Geriatric Otolaryngology

Editor

KAREN M. KOST

CLINICS IN
GERIATRIC MEDICINE

www.geriatric.theclinics.com

May 2018 • Volume 34 • Number 2

ELSEVIER

1600 John F. Kennedy Boulevard ● Suite 1800 ● Philadelphia, Pennsylvania, 19103-2899

http://www.theclinics.com

CLINICS IN GERIATRIC MEDICINE Volume 34, Number 2
May 2018 ISSN 0749–0690, ISBN-13: 978-0-323-58354-1

Editor: Jessica McCool
Developmental Editor: Laura Fisher

Clinics in Geriatric Medicine (ISSN 0749-0690) is published quarterly by Elsevier Inc., 360 Park Avenue South, New York, NY 10010-1710. Months of issue are February, May, August, and November. Business and Editorial Offices: 1600 John F. Kennedy Blvd., Suite 1800, Philadelphia, PA 191023-2899. Periodicals postage paid at New York, NY, and additional mailing offices. Subscription prices are $278.00 per year (US individuals), $602.00 per year (US institutions), $100.00 per year (US student/resident), $320.00 per year (Canadian individuals), $763.00 per year (Canadian institutions), $195.00 per year (Canadian student/resident), $402.00 per year (international individuals), $763.00 per year (international institutions), and $195.00 per year (international student/resident). Foreign air speed delivery is included in all *Clinics* subscription prices. All prices are subject to change without notice. POSTMASTER: Send address changes to *Clinics in Geriatric Medicine,* Elsevier Health Sciences Division, Subscription Customer Service, 3251 Riverport Lane, Maryland Heights, MO 63043. **Telephone: 1-800-654-2452 (U.S. and Canada); 314-447-8871 (outside U.S. and Canada). Fax: 314-447-8029. E-mail:** journalscustomerservice-usa@elsevier. com **(for print support) or** journalsonlinesupport-usa@elsevier.com **(for online support)**.

Reprints. For copies of 100 or more, of articles in this publication, please contact the Commercial Reprints Department, Elsevier Inc., 360 Park Avenue South, New York, New York 10010-1710. Tel.: 212-633-3874; Fax: 212-633-3820, E-mail: reprints@elsevier.com.

Clinics in Geriatric Medicine is covered in *MEDLINE/PubMed (Index Medicus), EMBASE/Excerpta Medica, Current Contents/Clinical Medicine (CC/CM),* and the *Cumulative Index to Nursing & Allied Health Literature.*

Contributors

EDITOR

KAREN M. KOST, MD, FRCSC
Professor of Otolaryngology–Head and Neck Surgery, Director of the Voice and Dysphagia Laboratory, McGill University, Montreal, Québec, Canada

AUTHORS

TAKUMI CODÈRE-MARUYAMA, MD, MSc
Assistant Professor, Department of Anesthesia, McGill University, Montreal, Québec, Canada

DAVID EIBLING, MD, FACS
Vice Chair for Education, Professor, Department of Otolaryngology–Head and Neck Surgery, University of Pittsburgh School of Medicine, Eye and Ear Institute, Staff Otolaryngologist, VA Pittsburgh Healthcare System, Assistant Chief of Surgery VA Pittsburgh, Pittsburgh, Pennsylvania, USA

KEVIN HIGGINS, MD, MSc, FACS, FRCSC
Department of Otolaryngology–Head and Neck Surgery, Sunnybrook Health Sciences Centre, Toronto, Ontario, Canada

BRIAN B. HUGHLEY, MD
Assistant Professor, Otolaryngology–Head and Neck Surgery, The University of Alabama at Birmingham, Birmingham, Alabama, USA

JONAS T. JOHNSON, MD, FACS
The Eugene N. Myers, MD, Professor and Chairman, Department of Otolaryngology, Professor, Department of Radiation Oncology, University of Pittsburgh School of Medicine, Eye and Ear Institute, Professor, Department of Oral and Maxillofacial Surgery, University of Pittsburgh School of Dental Medicine, Professor, Department of Communication Science and Disorders, School of Health and Rehabilitation Sciences, University of Pittsburgh, Pittsburgh, Pennsylvania, USA

KAREN M. KOST, MD, FRCSC
Professor of Otolaryngology–Head and Neck Surgery, Director of the Voice and Dysphagia Laboratory, McGill University, Montreal, Québec, Canada

LEILA J. MADY, MD, PhD, MPH
Postdoctoral Scholar, Department of Otolaryngology, University of Pittsburgh School of Medicine, Eye and Ear Institute, Pittsburgh, Pennsylvania, USA

BRIAN J. McKINNON, MD, MBA, MPH, FACS
Associate Professor and Vice Chair, Department of Otolaryngology–Head and Neck Surgery, Associate Professor, Department of Neurosurgery, Drexel University, College of Medicine, Philadelphia, Pennsylvania, USA

ALBERT MOORE, MD
Associate Professor, Department of Anesthesia, McGill University, Montreal, Québec, Canada

MARCI L. NILSEN, PhD, RN
Assistant Professor, Department of Acute and Tertiary Care, University of Pittsburgh School of Nursing, Pittsburgh, Pennsylvania, USA

ROHAN PATEL, BS
MD Candidate Class of 2018, Drexel University, College of Medicine, Philadelphia, Pennsylvania, USA

ROBERT T. SATALOFF, MD, DMA
Professor and Chairman, Department of Otolaryngology–Head and Neck Surgery, Senior Associate Dean for Clinical Academic Specialties, Drexel University, College of Medicine, Philadelphia, Pennsylvania, USA

CECELIA E. SCHMALBACH, MD, MS, FACS
Professor, Otolaryngology–Head and Neck Surgery, Division Chief, Head and Neck–Microvascular Surgery, Vice Chairman, Clinical Affairs, Indiana University School of Medicine, Indianapolis, Indiana, USA

MARC A. TEWFIK, MD, MSc, FRCSC
Department of Otolaryngology–Head and Neck Surgery, McGill University Health Center, Montreal, Québec, Canada

OZLEM E. TULUNAY-UGUR, MD
Department of Otolaryngology–Head and Neck Surgery, University of Arkansas for Medical Sciences, Little Rock, Arkansas, USA

CONSTANZA J. VALDÉS, MD
Department of Otolaryngology–Head and Neck Surgery, Hospital del Salvador, Universidad de Chile, Department of Otolaryngology–Head and Neck Surgery, Clínica Las Condes, Santiago, Chile

KATHLEEN YAREMCHUK, MD, MSA
Chairman, Department of Otolaryngology–Head and Neck Surgery, Henry Ford Hospital, Detroit, Michigan, USA

Contents

> Presbycusis, or age-related hearing loss (ARHL), is the result of physiologic and pathologic changes associated with advancing age. ARHL presents typically with a high-frequency hearing loss, which contributes to greater trouble hearing consonants within words. Consonants convey the bulk of meaning within a word, and this loss of linguistic information results in complaints associated with ARHL. Hearing aids and cochlear implants significantly improve the lives of older adults with hearing loss, in particular, those with depression and dementia. Successful current research in gene therapy, pharmacotherapy, and stems cells holds the promise of being able to restore native cochlear function.

> Balance disorders are common in the elderly and can lead to falls, with resultant severe morbidity and even mortality. Progressive loss of vestibular function begins in middle age and is affected by multiple disease processes. Polypharmacy affects many disease processes in the elderly, with balance function being one of the most susceptible. Evaluation of the older patient with a balance disorder is critical for the well-being of these patients, as it may drive intervention. This article reviews balance disorders often encountered in older patients and makes recommendations regarding education of nonotolaryngologists.

> Geriatric dysphagia is an unrecognized and underdiagnosed problem with significant morbidity and potential mortality. It requires diligence by the clinician and a team approach for successful management. Careful history taking is the key in the treatment of these patients and determines further workup, as well as treatment.

> Presbyphonia is more common than appreciated by most physicians, and it is associated with undesirable vocal characteristics such as hoarseness, weakness, breathiness, instability, and tremulousness. Hearing impairment in the patient or his or her friends, family, and associates exacerbates the problem, resulting in depression and social withdrawal, further

reducing quality of life. Moreover, voice weakness and instability are all too often misinterpreted as reflecting intellectual instability. Expert diagnosis, medical treatment, voice therapy and training, and occasionally surgery usually can maintain or restore vocal stability and "youth."

Medical care for elderly patients is often distinctly different from that of younger counterparts. This is no truer than in a thyroid disorder context, where patients are often asymptomatic and polypharmacy is a potential consideration. Understanding how treatment of these patients can deviate from common practices is an essential asset to any health care provider. This article sheds light on those deviations and addresses inherent complexities in caring for elderly patients in an effort to improve quality of care. Topics considered range from general anatomic challenges to underlying biochemistry to adjuvant therapy options and surveillance.

Geriatric patients undergoing surgery have a whole set of specific physiologic changes, perioperative needs, and postoperative complications. This article presents an overview of the basic concepts and the evolving challenges pertaining to the care of geriatric patients undergoing otolaryngologic procedures from the perspective of the anesthesiologist.

Frailty and polypharmacy commonly affect disease processes and treatment of patients with otolaryngologic disorders. Although the 2 concepts are well known to geriatricians, they often elude other physicians, including otolaryngologists. This article reviews the common manifestations likely to be encountered in otolaryngology patients, reviews frailty measures in surgical patients, and makes recommendations regarding education of nongeriatricians.

CLINICS IN GERIATRIC MEDICINE

ISSUE OF RELATED INTEREST

Otolaryngologic Clinics, August 2017 (Vol. 50, No. 4)
Multidisciplinary Approach to Head and Neck Cancer
Maie A. St. John, *Editor*
Available at: http://www.oto.theclinics.com

THE CLINICS ARE AVAILABLE ONLINE!
Access your subscription at:
www.theclinics.com

Preface

Geriatric Otolaryngology: Why It Matters

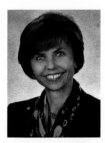

Karen M. Kost, MD, FRCSC
Editor

Historically, young children have always outnumbered older people. In what is a shifting global trend well known to the readers of this text, people over the age of 65 will, for the first time, soon outnumber children under the age of five. As a consequence of declining birth rates and increasing life spans, the geriatric age group is the fastest growing segment of our society.[1]

For some time, these shifting demographics have had a profound effect on medical and surgical subspecialties, including otolaryngology. Interestingly, the rise of geriatric otolaryngology as a firmly established subspecialty[2] is really the product of three major events. The first of these was the Geriatric Otolaryngology Cherry Blossom Conference held in Washington, DC in 1988. This meeting was attended by a number of visionary physicians, led by Jerome C. Goldstein, MD and resulted in the publication of a monograph entitled "Clinical Geriatric Otolaryngology." The second event was the Geriatrics for Specialists Initiative. Dr J. LoCicero, former chairman of the interspecialty group formed by the American Geriatric Society (AGS), understood that a crisis in elderly care was emerging. Over two decades ago, the AGS realized that it would need assistance in managing the increasing volume of geriatric patients and reached out to otolaryngology, among several specialties, to promote research and education within the subspecialty, and ultimately better prepare otolaryngologists to meet the evolving needs of the increasing elderly population. The third event was the birth of the American Society of Geriatric Otolaryngology in 2007, a result of the foresight and leadership of its first president, Jerome C. Goldstein, MD.

It is safe to say that elderly patients account for a disproportionately large and increasing number of outpatient visits to family physicians and otolaryngologists. As noted by Creighton and colleagues, the cross-section, or profile, of otolaryngologic pathologic conditions encountered in outpatient visits is not uniform across various age groups.[3] As this study demonstrated, otologic complaints are increasingly common

Clin Geriatr Med 34 (2018) ix–x
https://doi.org/10.1016/j.cger.2018.02.001
0749-0690/18/© 2018 Elsevier Inc. All rights reserved.

as patients age. The most common otolaryngologic diagnoses in patients over the age of 65, in order of frequency, were hearing loss, disorders of the external ear, "other" ear disorders consisting mainly of tinnitus, nonsuppurative otitis media/eustachian tube disorders, and vertiginous syndromes/vestibular disorders.[3] An awareness of the unique otolaryngologic pathologic condition profiles in geriatric patients is important in providing optimal care to this growing subset of the population. Moving forward, awareness of these important demographic changes in otolaryngology practices should translate into appropriate representation in training programs.

Functional abilities, independence, and a high quality of life feature prominently in the top priorities of geriatric patients and the physicians caring for them. Few would argue that hearing, taste, smell, and sensation are all senses that contribute, to an incalculable degree, to the sheer enjoyment, and quality, of life. The recognition that these senses are all part of the domain of Otolaryngology underscores the importance of this specialty in the elderly population.

Karen M. Kost, MD, FRCSC
McGill University Health Center
Room DS1-3310, 1001 Decarie Boulevard
Montreal, QC H4A 3J1, Canada

E-mail address:
kmkost@yahoo.com

REFERENCES

1. Shapiro DP. Geriatric demographics and the practice of otolaryngology. Ear Nose Throat J 1999;78(6):418–21.
2. Chalian A. Accomplishment and opportunity in geriatric otolaryngology. Ear Nose Throat J 2009;88(10):1156–61.
3. Creighton FX Jr, Poliashenko SM, Statham MM, et al. The growing geriatric otolaryngology patient population: a study of 131,700 new patient encounters. Laryngoscope 2013;123(1):97–102.

Hearing Loss in the Elderly

Rohan Patel, BS[a], Brian J. McKinnon, MD, MBA, MPH[b],*

KEYWORDS

- Elderly • Geriatrics • Age-related hearing loss • Presbycusis • Hearing aids
- Osseointegrated auditory implants • Cochlear implants • Regenerative therapies

KEY POINTS

- Hearing loss is a common sequela of aging and has a significant adverse impact on the health and well-being of the elderly.
- The hearing loss of aging reflects changes in both the peripheral and central auditory systems, with the greatest impact initially on the higher frequencies that are most important to understanding spoken language.
- Older patients, especially those with depression and dementia, benefit significantly from amplification and from cochlear implantation, although use of these technologies is not widespread within the population that could most benefit.
- There is a great deal of promising research focused on the regeneration of inner hair cells, in the areas of gene therapy, pharmacotherapy, and stem cells, that may in the near future markedly improve the lives of those with age-related hearing loss.

INTRODUCTION

Much like the advent of penicillin in 1928, advances in medical technology and health care have led to an increase in life expectancy with a steep rise in the numbers of older Americans. Population reports from the US Census Bureau indicate that the percentage of residents 65 and older grew from 12.4% (35 million) in 2000 to 15.2% (49.2 million) in 2016 with the national median age increasing from 35.3 years in 2000 to 37.9 years in 2016.[1] Life expectancy for those 65 years of age and older increased by 15.2 more years in 1972 and then to 19.1 more years in 2010. A similar trend is seen for individuals 85 and older, from 5.5 more years of life expectancy in 1972 to 6.5 more years of life expectancy in 2010. This is projected to continue with those 65 years and older predicted to have 20.6 more years of life expectancy and those 85 years and older having 7 more years of life expectancy by 2050.[2] This growth within

Disclosures: Neither author has disclosure of any relationship with a commercial company that has a direct financial interest in subject matter or materials discussed in article or with a company making a competing product.

[a] Drexel University College of Medicine, 2900 West Queen Lane, Philadelphia, PA 19129, USA;
[b] Departments of Otolaryngology–Head and Neck Surgery and Neurosurgery, 219 North Broad Street, 10th Floor, Philadelphia, PA 19107, USA
* Corresponding author. 219 North Broad Street, 10th Floor, Philadelphia, PA 19107.
E-mail address: bmckinnon@phillyent.com

the older population presupposes an associated increase in geriatric and degenerative issues. Alterations in sensory functions, vision, balance, and hearing are some of the most common disturbances seen in the aging population and lead to dramatic social and functional disability.

Among the senses affected by increasing age, hearing loss is the most common. Presbycusis, or age-related hearing loss (ARHL), is a term that refers to hearing loss as a result of physiologic and pathologic changes associated with increasing age. As the aging population continues to grow, greater focus is placed on understanding and attempting to reverse this sensory loss for the benefit of geriatric patients. Today, there is an established although still evolving concept of the workings of the outer ear, middle ear, and inner ear. This basis has led to a better understanding of aberrant behavior in both the peripheral and central auditory pathways, resulting in various forms of geriatric hearing loss. With a strong understanding of the foundation of geriatric hearing loss, more focused and novel areas of research are being investigated with promising results.

PRESENTATION

Presbycusis may present insidiously and be confounded by various medical, psychological, and pharmacologic factors. Only after thorough history, examination, and audiological testing can a diagnosis of presbycusis be made after excluding concurrent medical and pharmacologic effects. In general, the first signs of ARHL can be seen in late middle age with high-frequency hearing losses in the realm of conversation frequencies, ultimately progressing subtly to lower frequency tones. The range of human auditory frequencies spans 20 Hz to 20,000 Hz, with speech frequencies ranging from 400 Hz to 5000 Hz, with the greatest loss in hearing seen in frequencies greater than or equal to 2000 Hz.[3,4] The challenge to effortlessly understand speech stems from the natural frequencies of voice used to phonate consonants and vowels. In general, vowels vibrate at frequencies less than 1500 Hz compared with consonants, which vibrate at 1500 Hz or higher and are more softly spoken. Consequently, patients with ARHL have greater trouble hearing consonants within words that convey the bulk of the meaning within a word, are used to separate syllables, and indicate separation of words. The loss of this linguistic information results in many of the complaints in presbycusis. The loss of meaning is seen in deterioration of speech intelligibility, the loss of clear separation between words results in speech sounding mumbled, and the loss of syllables causes difficulty discerning similarly sounding words. Furthermore, similar to the natural frequencies of vowels and consonants, elderly patients may complain of difficulty hearing and understanding women and children, because their vocal registers are set to a higher range than are those for men. Patients with presbycusis rely on conversational, emotional, and postural context clues to compensate for their hearing impairment, requiring a greater amount of higher order cognitive functioning to understand daily conversations.

As the hearing loss progresses into lower frequencies, the difficulty becomes more apparent because a greater frequency range is affected and deficits are seen more often and in a greater number of conversations. Even if subconscious, the increased dependence on higher cognitive functioning to understand daily conversations puts the geriatric patient at increased strain when hearing in difficult hearing environments or with unfamiliar vocation. For example, conversations in noisy and crowded environments, such as restaurants and public areas, or with individuals with accents or faster speech result in a diminished speech intelligibility. As a product of relying on greater supplementary information to understand individual conversations, patients may seem aloof or inattentive, because they require a greater amount of time to process various information before being able to fully understand a conversation and respond appropriately. Patients having an incrementally difficult time hearing and understanding in these more complicated environments and dialogues are more likely to withdraw from future conversations in similar settings.

Of concern to older patients and their families is that alarm sounds, such as police sirens and fire alarms, sounds that are intended to keep people safe, use high-frequency sounds, which are difficult for this population to hear and recognize. Patients become a danger to themselves and others when they are not able to respond to a police car behind them or to a fire alarm going off in their apartment complexes. A study on sensory impairment and driving found that adults with right-sided hearing impairment were associated with increased risk in motor vehicle accidents in countries with right-sided steering wheels but concluded more studies need to be conducted to strengthen this finding.[5] This serious consequence of high-frequency sensorineural hearing loss is also compounded by difficulty in localizing sounds with age.[6] The effort to identify where a sound is originating from stems from an age-induced increase in neural temporal jitter of the central auditory processing system causing distorted representation of incoming sound.[7] This added complexity makes the ubiquitous use of high-frequency sounds not only a daily nuisance and social issue for the elderly hearing impaired population but also in some circumstances may put them in life-threatening danger.

Patients are forced to cope with the frustration of daily auditory difficulties, a response dependent on personal ability to manage stress. In general, patients may reflect the frustration externally or internally. Externally, patients may claim that their grandchildren mumble or speak too fast or too quietly. Internally, patients may isolate themselves and withdraw from conversations taking place right in front of them. This isolation may, in part, contribute to the delay in treatment of ARHL.

HEARING LOSS AND COGNITION

As discussed previously, hearing loss has a strong association with increased isolation and frustration. Not surprisingly, the reported prevalence of hearing loss in older adults with cognitive impairment is 60%.[8] Mounting evidence indicates that management of hearing loss is a key factor in the management of cognitive decline or dementia.[9] Although pharmacologic therapies for the management of dementia are available, patients with dementia also benefit from active social participation and engagement. The Memory–HEARS (Hearing Equality through Accessible Research Solutions) pilot study found that for the depression and neuropsychiatric outcome measures, participants with high symptom burden at baseline showed improvement at 1-month postintervention.[10] As noted in a recent review, however, hearing aid use has not been shown to improve cognitive function or slow the rate of cognitive decline.[11]

Addressing a hearing loss that impairs good communication is a requirement for a meaningful and engaging interaction and is a critical component of dementia care.[12,13] Hearing-impaired older adults who use hearing aids have a lower incidence of depression, and amplification also has a positive impact on hearing impaired older adults with depression. In older adults who used hearing aids or cochlear implants, there was a significant improvement in depressive symptoms at 6 months after treatment in those using cochlear implants and hearing aids and in those using cochlear implants the improvement persisted at 1 year.[14]

MANAGEMENT

Because patients with a hearing loss may not perceive themselves as having a hearing loss, it is important that those caring for older patients to ask about difficulty with communication and understanding conversation. Fewer than half of patients report being asked about hearing loss by their health care provider.[15] Hearing is assessed using pure-tone audiometry.[16] A pure tone of a specific frequency of increasing loudness is presented to 1 ear in a quiet setting until the sound intensity level at which it is perceived 50% of the time. This point is known as the pure-tone threshold for that ear at that frequency. Speech discrimination testing is performed once a patient's hearing thresholds have been established. The audiogram is a graphical display of those pure-tone thresholds as a function of frequency.[16]

In those older adults in whom a hearing loss is identified, consideration should be given to evaluation by a specialist. The following signs and symptoms should prompt evaluation by an otolaryngologist: pain, sudden-onset hearing loss, dizziness, ear deformity, burdensome or bothersome tinnitus, ear drainage, asymmetric hearing loss, unexplained conductive hearing loss, a history indicating ear infections, noise exposure, autoimmune disorder, ototoxic medication use, or otosclerosis, and visualization of blood, pus, cerumen, or foreign body in the ear canal.[17] In addition to the consideration of hearing aids, teaching communications strategies is important. Minimizing background noise, encouraging face-to-face interaction, and teaching patients to rephrase and summarize what they heard to ensure good comprehension are strategies that help with improving communication.[18]

HEARING AIDS

Medical evidence indicates that hearing aids improve the health-related quality of life by reducing the psychological, emotional, and social effects of hearing loss, particularly for older adults with mild to moderate hearing loss.[11] Improvement in health-related quality of life is seen in older adults who use a standard hearing aid, a programmable hearing aid with settings for different listening environments, or an assistive listening device. Despite marked improvements in hearing aid technology, according to 1 study, no improvements in hearing aid usage were noted over a 15-year period.[19,20]

Hearing aids may be analog or digital. Analog hearing aids are less expensive than digital hearing aids and work on a linear model of amplification, with a microphone collecting sound, the device converting the sound into an electrical signal and then amplifying the sound as it sends the sound through the canal to the tympanic membrane. Although both analog and digital hearing aids can be programmed for different listening conditions, digital hearing aids operate more automatically and adaptively, with programs that reduce acoustic feedback, reduce background noise, and detect and automatically accommodate different listening environments. Digital hearing aids are able to control additional components, such as multiple microphones, to improve spatial hearing, and, for example, transpose frequencies from where a user may have poor hearing to frequencies where the use may have better hearing.[21] Many current digital hearing aids can also connect, or pair, with cell phones, digital music devices, and other electronic devices, allowing for a markedly improved hearing experience.

OSSEOINTEGRATED AUDITORY IMPLANTS

Osseointegrated auditory implants like the bone-anchored hearing aid (BAHA) systems are approved in the United States for patients with single-sided deafness

(SSD) or those with a conductive/mixed hearing loss (CMHL) who cannot use traditional amplification. The use of BAHA systems began in patients with dental implants. These individuals noted the perception of sound through an osseointegrated dental implant. With the advances in BAHA technology and technique, complications have been minimized and are generally minor.[22]

BAHA systems use an external processor to amplify sound waves as vibrations that are delivered to the inner ear. For patients with CMHL, the amplification involves bypassing the external canal and middle ear and using bone conduction to transmit sound energy to the ipsilateral cochlea.[23] For patients with SSD/unilateral sensorineural hearing loss, auditory information is transmitted to the contralateral cochlea.[24] In patients with SSD/CMHL, BAHA systems can provide hearing improvements that are not possible with conventional hearing aids alone, because conventional aids only amplify sound, and they must use the natural conducting mechanism of the outer ear and middle ear.[25] As a result, they have become an attractive alternative to traditional hearing aids in select older patients.

Older patients fitted with a BAHA experience substantially improved hearing and word and speech recognition and obtain greater sound localization, and substantial numbers report improvement in quality of life as measured by instruments, such as as the Glasgow Benefit Inventory,[26] a validated instrument used to assess the benefit of amplification.[27] The most common adverse event is skin reaction, including hypertrophic scarring and generalized irritation, with poor osseointegration and implant failure overall rare but reportedly more common in older populations.[25]

COCHLEAR IMPLANTATION

Although most older patients are appropriate candidates for amplification, up to 10% of older patients with hearing loss suffer from hearing loss severe enough that amplification cannot provide significant benefit.[28] Cochlear implants, devices placed into the inner ear to restore the perception of sound, are an effective intervention for older patients who do not benefit from amplification. Unfortunately, the rate of cochlear implant use in older adults who meet candidacy criteria is less than 5%.[29] Outcomes of cochlear implantation are closely related to the duration of deafness, and counseling patients and their families on reasonable expectations is essential. Cognitive evaluations can help guide assessment and counseling.[30]

Because a detailed description of cochlear implantation in the older patient can be found elsewhere,[31] a brief description follows. Cochlear implantation is a surgery commonly performed under general anesthesia, lasting less than 2 hours. Despite the short nature of the surgery, careful attention must be paid to medical comorbidities.[31] Medical optimization and clearance by patients' primary care provider and other specialists, as appropriate, is prudent to ensure a safe procedure and successful recovery. Older patients on anticoagulation therapy should obtain recommendations from the prescribing physician on how to best bridge the perioperative period. Cochlear implantation in older patients is safe and without significant risk in medically optimized individuals,[32,33] with no perioperative deaths having been reported.[34–36] Significant postoperative pain or nausea is rarely encountered and less common in older adults than in younger adults,[37] with older patients frequently returning to their normal routine within days.

Postoperative rehabilitation in older patients is similar to that in other adult patients, with speech perception testing the most important guide for rehabilitation. As noted in a review of current postoperative audiological and quality-of-life findings, there are several measures and instruments used to assess the audiological and quality-of-life outcomes achieved by geriatric cochlear implant recipients.[38] Geriatric cochlear implant users enjoy improved speech perception and have outcomes for speech perception in a quiet environment comparable to other cochlear implant users, although younger postlingual cochlear implant users have better speech perception in noise than older cochlear implant users. This differences may reflect a longer duration of hearing loss and poorer preoperative speech perception. Older patients tend to have a somewhat slower rate of speech perception gain, and there is strong correlation between length of daily cochlear implant use and speech perception performance. When preoperative speech perception was taken into account, age was not predictive of postoperative speech perception outcome.[31,37]

Unilateral older and younger cochlear implant users report a similar speech perception benefit, but bilateral older cochlear implant users report less speech perception benefit than either unilateral older or younger cochlear implant users.[37] Many older cochlear implant users report difficulty with telephone conversation and conversation in noise and groups, although larger speech perception gains are reported in those with increased social activity. Speech perception achievements seem stable over the long term and may continue to improve.[37,38] Older cochlear implant users show greater confidence and participation in social settings than they did preoperatively. Moreover, older cochlear implant users and their families also reported high levels of satisfaction and hearing benefits from their devices.

Because Medicare uses candidate criteria that are significantly more restrictive than those set forward by the Food and Drug Administration,[39] and because preoperative speech perception is an important predictor of postoperative success, this likely skews the outcomes data, leading to under-representation of the benefit for older patients in whom amplification cannot help. In terms of economic efficacy, geriatric cochlear implantation compares favorably with pediatric and adult cochlear implantation, despite shorter life expectancy.[40] The rates of long-term use and nonuse also compare favorably with children and adult cochlear implant recipients.[41,42] Access challenges to funding and reimbursement are relevant to older patients. According to a RAND Corporation–funded study reviewing payments received for cochlear implants by providers and facilities in the United States, a hospital faced an average loss of $5000 to $10,000 on every Medicare patient implanted, making the provision of cochlear implantation to geriatric candidates economically tenuous.[43,44]

Taken together, the lack of adequate reimbursement and the restrictive candidate criteria risk reduced access to cochlear implantation for many geriatric patients who could benefit.

REGENERATIVE THERAPIES

With an increasing number of patients afflicted by presbycusis, greater attention is focused on novel therapies for treatment of ARHL. Hearing aids, BAHAs, and cochlear implants do not help regain native cochlear function or reverse any of the damage to the cochlear hair cells. ARHL is due in part to the loss of cochlear inner hair cells, which are responsible for the mechanosensory transmission of vibratory frequencies into neural input. There has been a significant interest in methods to regenerate cochlear inner hair cells since a study in 1993 found regeneration of inner ear sensory hair cells within the vestibular sensory epithelium of adult guinea pigs and humans.[45] Current research is focused on the usefulness of gene therapy, stem cell use, and pharmaceuticals to jump start the regeneration of inner hair cells.

GENE THERAPY

Of particular interest to hearing loss has been the role of the Atoh1 transcription factor, which has been found to play a crucial role in the differentiation of cochlear and vestibular hair cells.[46] Atoh1 expression leads to the formation of sensory hair cells and also to neurogenesis and functional inner ear hair cells.[47–50] Cell-cycle modulators is another area of gene therapy being targeted to enhance and tailor the regeneration of hair cells. p27[Kip1] is a cyclin-dependent kinase inhibitor seen to maintain quiescence of supporting cells and coincides with cell-cycle exit of hair cell and supporting cell progenitors.[51–55] Further work has established safe nondamaging administrative methods for gene therapy and future potential stem cell and pharmacologic therapies.[56]

PHARMACOTHERAPY

Closely linked with gene transcription and downstream effects are cellular signaling pathways and molecules, 2 of the most investigated pathways being the Wnt and Notch signaling cascades. Both are implicated in cellular proliferation and differentiation, whereas Wnt also regulates cellular migration, polarity, and neural patterning, and Notch regulates cellular patterning and apoptosis.[57–63] It has been shown that Notch signaling cascade promotes supporting cell transdifferentiation to regenerate hair cells rather than proliferation, slowly exhausting the population of supporting cells. Furthermore, Wnt activation results in a greater proliferation of supporting cells but a limited growth of hair cells.[64–66]

STEM CELLS

Although some researchers have reported success with hair cell–like cells from mouse embryonic stem cells and induced pluripotent stem cells,[67] others have focused on the development of the neural component of the inner ear system.[68] Several studies have shown success with mesenchymal stem cells in regenerating cochlear spiral ganglion neurons and restoration of some improved auditory brainstem response and otoacoustic emission.[69–71] Work with endogenous stem cells could bypass some challenges of exogenous stem cell use, with the best source for use in hearing restoration under investigation.[72–76]

SUMMARY

Geriatric hearing loss is a byproduct of normal aging with serious implications on individual and public social health and safety. Hearing loss is often an unrecognized concern in older patients with depression and dementia. Management of hearing loss through hearing aids and cochlear implantation has short-term and long-term benefits to quality of life, improving mood and social interaction. Amplification should be combined with the teaching of listening skills to help facilitate communication. Osseointegrated auditory implants and cochlear implantation are important surgical options for those who may not benefit from conventional hearing aids. Cochlear implantation is performed under general anesthesia and is safe and well tolerated by older adults, and older adults perform postoperatively similarly to younger adult cochlear implant patients. Hearing aids and cochlear implants do not prevent or repair the underlying pathophysiology of ARHL. Interest in inner ear regenerative therapies with hopes for more definitive treatment have made significant advancements since interest in the area first grew but still faces many challenges. Among these common hurdles is that each regenerative approach possesses unique advantages and challenges that in time may be overcome and provide innovative methods to treat geriatric hearing loss.

REFERENCES

1. Newcomb A, Iriondo J. The nation's older population is still growing, census bureau reports. Washington, DC: United States Census Bureau; 2017. Available at: https://www.census.gov/newsroom/press-releases/2017/cb17-100.html. Accessed October 29, 2017.
2. Ortman J, Velkoff V, Hogan H. An aging nation: the older population in the United States. Washington, DC: United States Census Bureau; 2014. Available at: https://www.census.gov/prod/2014pubs/p25-1140.pdf. Accessed October 29, 2017.
3. Martin FN, Clack JG. Introduction to audiology. 8th edition. Needham Heights (MA): Allyn & Bacon; 2003.
4. Humes LE, Burk MH, Strauser LE, et al. Development and efficacy of a frequent-word auditory training protocol for older adults with impaired hearing. Ear Hear 2009;30(5):613–27.
5. Ivers RQ, Mitchell P, Cumming RG. Sensory impairment and driving: the blue mountains eye study. Am J Public Heath 1999;89(1):85–7.
6. Abel SM, Giguère C, Consoli A, et al. The effect of aging on horizontal plane sound localization. J Acoust Soc Am 2000;108(2):743–52.
7. Freigang C, Schmiedchen K, Nitsche I, et al. Freefield study on auditory localization and discrimination performance in older adults. Exp Brain Res 2014;232(4): 1157–72.
8. Nirmalasari O, Mamo SK, Nieman CL, et al. Age-related hearing loss in older adults with cognitive impairment. Int Psychogeriatr 2017;29(1):115–21.
9. Mamo SK, Oh E, Lin FR. Enhancing communication in adults with dementia and age-related hearing loss. Semin Hear 2017;38(2):177–83.
10. Mamo SK, Nirmalasari O, Nieman CL, et al. Hearing care intervention for persons with dementia: a pilot study. Am J Geriatr Psychiatry 2017;25(1):91–101.
11. Bainbridge KE, Wallhagen MI. Hearing loss in an aging American population: extent, impact, and management. Annu Rev Public Health 2014;35:139–52.
12. Cohen-Mansfield J, Dakheel-Ali M, Marx MS, et al. Which unmet needs contribute to behavior problems in persons with advanced dementia? Psychiatry Res 2015; 228(1):59–64.
13. Cohen-Mansfield J. Nonpharmacologic interventions for inappropriate behaviors in dementia: a review, summary, and critique. Am J Geriatr Psychiatry 2001;9(4): 361–81.
14. Choi JS, Betz J, Li L, et al. Association of using hearing aids or cochlear implants with changes in depressive symptoms in older adults. JAMA Otolaryngol Head Neck Surg 2016;142(7):652–7.
15. Kochkin S. MarkeTrak VII: obstacles to adult non- user adoption of hearing aids. Hearing J 2007;60(4):27–43.
16. Bagai A, Thavendiranathan P, Detsky AS. Does this patient have hearing impairment? JAMA 2006;295:416–28.
17. American Academy of Otolaryngology–Head and Neck Surgery. Position statement: red flags - warning of ear disease. 2014. Available at: http://www.entnet.org/content/red-flags-warning-ear-disease. Accessed December 9, 2017.
18. Contrera KJ, Wallhagen MI, Mamo SK, et al. Hearing loss health care for older adults. J Am Board Fam Med 2016;29(3):394–403.

19. Nash SD, Cruickshanks KJ, Huang GH, et al. Unmet hearing health care needs: the Beaver Dam offspring study. Am J Public Health 2013;103:1134–9.
20. Popelka M, Cruickshanks KJ, Wiley TL, et al. Low prevalence of hearing aid use among older adults with hearing loss: the epidemiology of hearing loss study. J Am Geriatr Soc 1998;46:1075–8.
21. Sprinzl GM, Riechelmann H. Current trends in treating hearing loss in elderly people: a review of the technology and treatment options - a mini-review. Gerontology 2010;56(3):351–8.
22. Badran K, Arya AK, Bunstone D, et al. Long-term complications of bone-anchored hearing aids: a 14-year experience. J Laryngol Otol 2009;123(2): 170–6.
23. Hol MK, Bosman AJ, Snik AF, et al. Bone-anchored hearing aids in unilateral inner ear deafness: an evaluation of audiometric and patient outcome measurements. Otol Neurotol 2005;26(5):999–1006.
24. Linstrom CJ, Silverman CA, Yu GP. Efficacy of the bone- anchored hearing aid for single-sided deafness. Laryngoscope 2009;119(4):713–20.
25. Dun CAJ, de Wolf MJF, Hol MKS, et al. Stability, survival, and tolerability of a novel baha implant system: six-month data from a multicenter clinical investigation. Otol Neurotol 2011;32(6):1001–7.
26. Faber HT, de Wold MJ, Cremers CW, et al. Benefit of BAHA in the elderly with single sided deafness. Eur Arch Otorhinolaryngol 2013;270(4):1285–91.
27. Gatehouse S. Glasgow hearing aid benefit profile: derivation and validation of a client-centered outcome measure for hearing-aid services. J Am Acad Audiol 1999;10:80–103.
28. Havlik RJ. Aging in the eighties, impaired senses for sound and light in persons age 65 years and over. Adv Data 1986;125:1–7.
29. Lin FR. Hearing loss and cognition among older adults in the United States. J Gerontol A Biol Sci Med Sci 2011;66(10):1131–6.
30. Rossi-Katz J, Arehart KH. Survey of audiologic service provision to older adults with cochlear implants. Am J Audiol 2011;20(2):84–9.
31. Coelho DH, McKinnon BJ. Cochlear implants in the geriatric population. In: Sataloff RT, Johns MM, Kost KM, editors. Geriatric otolaryngology. 1st edition. New York: Theime; 2015. p. 85–9.
32. Coelho DH, Yeh J, Lalwani AK. Cochlear implantation is associated with minimal anesthetic risk in the elderly. Laryngoscope 2009;119(2):355–8.
33. Carlson ML, Breen JT, Gifford RH, et al. Cochlear implantation in the octogenarian and nonagenarian. Otol Neurotol 2010;31(8):1343–9.
34. Chatelin V, Kim EJ, Driscoll C, et al. Cochlear implant outcomes in the elderly. Otol Neurotol 2004;25(3):298–301.
35. Alice B, Silvia M, Laura G, et al. Cochlear implantation in the elderly: surgical and hearing outcomes. BMC Surg 2013;13(Suppl 2):S1.
36. Sinclair DR, Chung F, Mezei G. Can postoperative nausea and vomiting be predicted? Anesthesiology 1999;91(1):109–18.
37. Clark JH, Yeagle J, Arbaje AI, et al. Cochlear implant rehabilitation in older adults: literature review and proposal of a conceptual framework. J Am Geriatr Soc 2012; 60(10):1936–45.
38. Dillon MT, Buss E, Adunka MC, et al. Long-term speech perception in elderly cochlear implant users. JAMA Otolaryngol Head Neck Surg 2013;139(3): 279–83.
39. Centers for Medicare and Medicaid Services. Medicare Benefit Policy Manual. Decision Memo for Cochlear Implantation (CAG-00107N). 2005. Available at: https://

www.cms.gov/medicare-coverage-database/details/ncd-details.aspx?NCDId=
245&ncdver=2&NCAId=134&DocID=CAG-00107N&generalError=Thank+you
+for+your+interest+in+the+Medicare+Coverage+Database.+You+may+only+
view+the+page+you+attempted+to+access+via+normal+usage+of+the+
Medicare+Coverage+Database.&bc=gAAAABAACAAAAA%3d%3d&. Accessed
December 10, 2017.

40. Francis HW, Chee N, Yeagle J, et al. Impact of cochlear implants on the functional
    health status of older adults. Laryngoscope 2002;112(8 Pt 1):1482–8.

41. Contrera KJ, Choi JS, Blake CR, et al. Rates of long-term cochlear implant use in
    children. Otol Neurotol 2014;35(3):426–30.

42. Bhatt YM, Green KM, Mawman DJ, et al. Device nonuse among adult cochlear
    implant recipients. Otol Neurotol 2005;26(2):183–7.

43. Garber S, Ridgely MS, Bradley M, et al. Payment under public and private insur-
    ance and access to cochlear implants. Arch Otolaryngol Head Neck Surg 2002;
    128(10):1145–52.

44. McKinnon BJ. Cochlear implant programs: balancing clinical and financial sus-
    tainability. Laryngoscope 2013;123(1):233–8.

45. Wharcol ME, Lambert PR, Goldstein BJ, et al. Regenerative proliferation in inner
    ear sensory epithelia from adult guinea pigs and humans. Science 1993;
    259(5101):1619–22.

46. Birmingham NA, Hassan BA, Price SD, et al. Math1: an essential gene for the
    generation of inner ear hair cells. Science 1999;284(5421):1837–41.

47. Kawamoto K, Ishimoto S, Minoda R, et al. Math1 gene transfer generates
    new cochlear hair cells in mature guinea pigs in vivo. J Neurosci 2003;23(11):
    4395–400.

48. Izumikawa M, Minoda R, Kawamoto K, et al. Auditory hair cell replacement and
    hearing improvement by Atoh1 gene therapy in deaf mammals. Nat Med 2005;
    11(3):271–6.

49. Mahmoodian sani MR, Hashemzadeh-Chaleshtori M, Saidijam M, et al. MicroRNA-
    183 family in inner ear: hair cell development and deafness. J Audiol Otol 2016;
    20(3):131–8.

50. Ebeid M, Sripal P, Pecka J, et al. Transcriptome-wide comparison of the Atoh1
    and miR-183 family on pluripotent stem cells and multipotent otic progenitor cells.
    PLoS One 2017;12(7):e0180855.

51. Lee YS, Liu F, Segil N. A morphogenic wave of p27Kip1 transcription directs cell
    cycle exit during organ of Corti development. Development 2006;133(15):
    2817–36.

52. Lowenheim H, Furness DN, Kil J, et al. Gene disruption of p27(Kip1) allows cell
    proliferation in the postnatal and adult organ of corti. Proc Natl Acad Sci U S A
    1999;96(7):4084–8.

53. Walters BJ, Liu Z, Crabtree M, et al. Auditory hair cell-specific deletion of p27Kip1
    in postnatal mice promotes cell-autonomous generation of new hair cells and
    normal hearing. J Neurosci 2014;34(47):15751–63.

54. Maass JC, Berndt FA, Canovas J, et al. P27Kip1 knockdown induces proliferation
    in the organ of Corti in culture after efficient shRNA lentiviral transduction. J Assoc
    Res Otolaryngol 2013;14(4):495–508.

55. Walters BJ, Coak E, Dearman J, et al. In vivo interplay between p27Kip1, GATA3,
    ATOH1, and POU4F3 converts non-sensory cells to hair cells in adult mice. Cell
    Rep 2017;19(2):307–20.

56. Chenkai D, Lehar M, Sun DQ, et al. Rhesus cochlear and vestibular functions are preserved after inner ear injection of saline volume sufficient for gene therapy delivery. J Assoc Res Otolaryngol 2017;18(4):601–17.
57. Logan CY, Nusse R. The Wnt signaling pathway in development and disease. Annu Rev Cell Dev Biol 2004;20(1):781–810.
58. Aster JC. Notch signalling in health and disease. J Pathol 2014;232(1):1–3.
59. Head JR, Gacioch L, Pennisi M, et al. Activation of canonical Wnt/β-catenin signaling stimulates proliferation in neuromasts in the zebrafish posterior lateral line. Dev Dyn 2013;242(7):832–46.
60. Shi F, Kempfle JS, Edge AS. Wnt-responsive Lgr5-expressing stem cells are hair cell progenitors in the cochlea. J Neurosci 2012;32(28):9639–48.
61. Shi2 F, Cheng YF, Wang XL, et al. β-catenin up-regulates Atoh1 expression in neural progenitor cells by interaction with an Atoh1 3′ enhancer. J Biol Chem 2010;285(1):392–400.
62. Korrapati S, Roux I, Glowatzki E, et al. Notch signaling limits supporting cell plasticity in the hair cell-damaged early postnatal murine cochlea. PLoS One 2013; 8(8):e73276.
63. Mizutari K, Fujioka M, Hosoya M, et al. Notch inhibition induces cochlear hair cell regeneration and recovery of hearing after acoustic trauma. Neuron 2013;77(1): 58–69.
64. Ni W, Zeng S, Li W, et al. Wnt activation followed by Notch inhibition promotes mitotic hair cell regeneration in the postnatal mouse cochlea. Oncotarget 2016; 7(41):66754–68.
65. Wu J, Li W, Lin C, et al. Co-regulation of the notch and wnt signaling pathways promotes supporting cell proliferation and hair cell regeneration in mouse utricles. Sci Rep 2016;6:29418.
66. Munnamalai V, Fekete DM. Notch-Wnt-Bmp crosstalk regulates radial patterning in the mouse cochlea in a spatiotemporal manner. Development 2016;143(21): 4003–15.
67. Oshima K, Shin K, Diesthuber M, et al. Mechanosensitive hair cell-like cells from embryonic and induced pluripotent stem cells. Cell 2010;141(4): 704–16.
68. Matsuoka AJ, Morrissey ZD, Zhang C, et al. Directed differentiation of human embryonic stem cells toward placode-derived spiral ganglion-like sensory neurons. Stem Cells Transl Med 2017;6(3):923–36.
69. Bas E, Van Der Water TR, Lumbreras V, et al. Adult human nasal mesenchymal-like stem cells restore cochlear spiral ganglion neurons after experimental lesion. Stem Cells Dev 2014;23(5):502–14.
70. Jang S, Cho H, Kim S, et al. Neural-induced human mesenchymal stem cells promote cochlear cell regeneration in deaf guinea pigs. Clin Exp Otorhinolaryngol 2015;8(2):83–91.
71. Kil K, Choi MY, Kong JS, et al. Regenerative efficacy of mesenchymal stromal cells from human placenta in sensorineural hearing loss. Int J Pediatr Otorhinolaryngol 2016;91:72–81.
72. Oshima K, Grimm CM, Corrales E, et al. Differential distribution of stem cells in the auditory and vestibular organs of the inner ear. J Assoc Res Otolaryngol 2007;8(1):18–31.
73. Lou X, Xie J, Wang X, et al. Comparison of sphere-forming capabilities of the cochlear stem cells derived from the apical, middle, basal turns of murine organ of corti. Neurosci Lett 2014;579:1–6.

74. Watanabe R, Morell MH, Miller JM, et al. Nestin-expressing cells in the developing, mature and noise-exposed cochlear epithelium. Mol Cell Neurosci 2012; 49(2):104–9.

75. Taniguchi M, Yamamoto N, Nakagawa T, et al. Identification of tympanic border cells as slow-cycling cells in the cochlea. PLoS One 2012;7(10): e48544.

76. Smeti I, Savary E, Capelle V, et al. Expression of candidate markers for stem/progenitor cells in the inner ears of developing and adult GFAP and nestin promoter-GFP transgenic mice. Gene Expr Patterns 2011;11(1–2):22–32.

Balance Disorders in Older Adults

David Eibling, MD

KEYWORDS

- Falls • Balance disorders • Presbystasis • Dizziness • Vestibular disorders • Frailty
- Polypharmacy

KEY POINTS

- Vestibular function begins to decrease in middle age.
- Benign paroxysmal positional vertigo (BPPV) is the most common cause of vertigo in elderly.
- Balance disorders in the elderly are rarely caused by vestibular disease.
- Many medications affect balance and contribute to falls.
- Intervention for balance disorders should focus on reducing the number of medications, environmental enhancements, and vestibular rehabilitation.

INTRODUCTION

Balance disorders are common in older adults, and may lead to substantial morbidity by increasing the risk for falls (**Box 1**). It has been estimated that as many as one-third of older adults may suffer some complaint interpreted as dizziness in a typical year. Lin and Bhattacharyya reported on data on 37 million surveyed individuals 65 years of age or older derived from the 2008 National Health Interview.[1] Nineteen percent reported they had experienced dizziness or balance disorders in the past year. Of this subset, 68% had suffered imbalance, 30% true vertigo, and nearly 30% complained of faintness. A little more than a quarter of the affected individuals (27%) had limited their activities because of their dizziness or imbalance.

Those individuals with true vertigo can be assumed to suffer from true vestibular diseases such as benign paroxysmal positional vertigo (BPPV), which will be discussed later. Those who experience faintness may have postural hypotension, which patients often report as dizziness. The majority, 68% in this cohort, can be assumed to have disorders of balance, or disequilibrium.

Agrawal and colleagues reported findings from a simple screening test performed on more than 5000 adults older than 40 who participated in the 2001 to 2004 National Health and Nutrition Examination Survey.[2] Subjects were asked to

The author has nothing to disclose.
Department of Otolaryngology–Head and Neck Surgery, VA Pittsburgh Healthcare System, University Drive C, Pittsburgh, PA 15240, USA
E-mail address: eiblingde@upmc.edu

Box 1
Causes of balance disorders

Vestibular
  Presbystasis
  Benign paroxysmal positional vertigo
  Meniere disease
  Vestibular neuronitis
  Vertibro-basilar insufficiency
  Postlabrynthitis vestibulopathy
  Migranous vertigo

Nonvestibular
  Frailty
  Multisensory disequilibrium
  Medications
    Sedative
    Psychoactive
    Anticholinergics
    Antihypertensives

---

stand on foam rubber with their eyes closed (modified Rhomberg on a compliant surface). More than a third (35%) had objective evidence of imbalance, and nearly one-half of adults in their 60s failed the test. Nearly 85% of the cohort 80 and older failed.

The figures quoted from Lin and Bhattacharyya add up to more than 100%, which is not surprising, since the complaint of dizziness can be attributed to a single diagnosis in less than one-half of affected patients. As in many other ailments affecting older adults, dizziness is typically multifactorial when encountered in the elderly. It is not uncommon to identify older adult patients presenting to an otolaryngologist with complaints of dizziness who have baseline presbystasis, episodic BPPV, orthostatic hypotension caused by antihypertensive medications, and exacerbation of their baseline presbystasis due to medications.

Despite the prevalence of balance disorders, affected individuals benefit from a comprehensive search for modifiable underlying etiologies. Many of these etiologies are well recognized by the readers of this article, but are often not apparent to practitioners without the benefit of training in gerontology. The role of the geriatric specialist in the education of primary care providers (PCPs) and other nongeriatricians is clear, particularly when sharing in the management of older adults who have balance disorders.

FALLS

The readers of this article need no reminding of the morbidity associated with balance disorders in older adults. The risk of falls in older adults is substantial, and increases dramatically with age and comorbidities. Recognition of the morbidity inherent in falls is not restricted to those who manage geriatric patients, or even to general health care workers. In fact, most individuals without medical training are aware of an older adult in their social circle who suffered a serious fall due to a balance disorder. An older family member of the author succumbed to a fall-induced closed head injury the day prior to starting this article, placing the significance of the issue in sharp focus.

The 2010 American Geriatric Society/British Geriatric Society (AGS/BGS) Clinical Practice Guideline (CPG) on fall prevention addresses the issue of falls in some detail. The themes of the CPG will be repeated and emphasized later in this article. This CPG should be read by all who manage older adults, not only by geriatricians.[3] Some estimate of the prevalence of balance disorders and the significance of the CPG can be deduced from the reports by Lin and Agrawal noted earlier.[1,2] Although balance function is not the only factor affecting fall risk, it clearly is among the most significant.

A common fallacy is to attribute all balance disorders to disorders of the vestibular system itself, when multiple systems are often responsible, primarily the peripheral nervous system and the musculoskeletal system. Otolaryngologists are often consulted for dizziness in elderly patients who do not have classic vestibulopathy. Evaluation will often demonstrate that the complaints stem from presbystasis, often aggravated by overmedication, or orthostatic hypotension caused by antihypertensive medications, rather than true vertigo.

PHYSIOLOGY OF THE AGING VESTIBULAR SYSTEM

Gradual degradation of vestibular function begins in midlife, but is not recognizable in its initial stages due to effective compensation. Normal aging is accompanied by loss of hair cells, fragmentation of otoconia, reduction of numbers of cells in the vestibular nuclei, and loss of afferent fibers. Slowing of motor responses and the progressive muscle loss of sarcopenia, along with other aliments accompanying frailty, reduce the ability of the older person to maintain an upright posture. Vestibular function decrement during the normal aging processes occurs symmetrically, and usually does not prompt investigation until some specific event. Routine vestibular testing, such as caloric testing, relies on comparison of right and left vestibular contributions and will fail to demonstrate degradation caused by symmetric changes. More sophisticated testing utilizing posturography, which seeks to isolate vestibular input by reducing or eliminating the compensatory contributions of proprioception and vision, is more effective in elucidating vestibular loss. More discrete identification of vestibular loss can be determined by rotational chair testing, which utilizes motion rather than caloric stimulation to assess vestibular effect on extraocular muscle activity (vestibular-ocular reflex, VOR). Other sophisticated testing such as vestibular evoked myogenic potentials (VEMPs) demonstrate elevated thresholds and reduced amplitude accompanying increasing age but are typically not helpful in clinical management of the aging vestibular system.[4]

When encountered clinically, the end result of these changes is described as presbystasis. Slowing of vestibular response to motion may be manifested by delay in moving from a sitting position to standing upright. Other phenotypic manifestations of presbystasis include slowing gait, reduced response to sudden motion, and inability to recover from a minor trip or misplaced foot. Although typically associated with multiple comorbidities, a recent review suggests that genetic factors may play a role in progression of balance disorders in the elderly.[5]

VESTIBULAR CAUSES OF BALANCE DISORDERS

Balance disorders in older adults can be roughly differentiated into vestibular and nonvestibular causes. It is usually possible to identify more than one etiologic entity, (eg, presbystasis and BPPV). With the exception of BPPV, classic vestibulopathies presenting with vertigo such as Meniere disease or vestibular neuritis are infrequently encountered in the elderly. Of elderly patients presenting with complaints of true vertigo, which is best described as "an illusion of motion," most will be found to be experiencing symptoms of BPPV.

BENIGN PAROXYSMAL POSITIONAL VERTIGO

As noted previously, the most common vestibulopathy affecting the elderly is BPPV. The descriptive term describes it well: episodes of true vertigo that is benign, brought on by position changes, and occur paroxysmally, often for several weeks before spontaneous resolution. Placing the patient in the precipitating position (Dix-Hallpike maneuver) leads to a 10- to 20-second episode of true vertigo with obvious nystagmus that follows a brief (2- to 5-second) latency, and resolves in less than a minute. This disorder accounts for approximately 10% of all cases of dizziness, and is easily diagnosed and treated. The reader is referred to the multiple descriptions if unfamiliar with the disorder. The CPG published by the American Academy of Otolaryngology–Head and Neck Surgery in 2008 was recently updated and is available online.[6] With the introduction of otolith repositioning by Epley in 1991, management is now easily performed by any provider or family member, and many patients perform self-repositioning when symptomatic. Widespread dissemination of the otolith repositioning procedure in several formats, including You Tube, has further eased the management of this common disorder and can be reviewed in real-time during patient encounters. The author typically recommends that his patients first view one of the many You Tube videos prior to returning to the clinic for repeat otolith repositioning.

MENIERE DISEASE

Most patients with Meniere disease have a long history of the typical syndrome of episodic severe vertigo accompanied by a sense of fullness in the ear, increase in tinnitus, and hearing loss. The reader is referred to the many excellent texts for further discussion of this disorder. Roughly 15% of cases of Meniere disease present initially in older patients. Long-standing Meniere disease in the elderly is typically accompanied by substantial hearing loss (in addition to the classic fluctuating loss associated with attack), hence the impact of further hearing loss, which can accompany labyrinthine ablation with intratympanic gentamycin is less severe should such become necessary. Occasionally patients with Meniere disease develop sudden drop attacks, sudden unpredictable falls that occur without a prodrome or loss of consciousness. These are termed "Tumarkin's otolithic crises," tend to occur in groups, and usually resolve spontaneously after about a year. When occurring in the elderly, they carry the additional risk of fracture.

POSTLABYRINTHITIS VESTIBULOPATHY

This disorder occurs as a sequela of a prior vestibular insult such as acute labyrinthitis, vascular compromise of the labyrinthine end-organ, or surgical or traumatic injury to the vestibular organ or its efferent neural pathways. Symptoms stem from asymmetrical input following resolution of the acute phase, and although theoretically a vestibular disorder, it typically presents more as a momentary disequilibrium precipitated by head motion. The condition is an unavoidable consequence of vestibular sacrifice such as from labyrinthine ablation, vestibular nerve section, or acoustic neuroma resection. Therapy is similar to presbystasis, avoidance of psychoactive medications and vestibular rehabilitation.

POLYPHARMACY

The statistics regarding the role of overmedication in precipitating or aggravating diseases in the elderly are staggering, and well known to the readership of this article. Disruption of balance function and precipitation of falls may be the greatest impact of overmedication for populations and individual patients. The AGS/BGS 2010 CPG on falls includes a detailed review of the literature supporting the connection between polypharmacy and falls, and the reader is referred to this document for more information. The CPG lists as its second recommendation "reduction of medications, especially psychoactive medications."[3] Often more than one drug class is responsible. A safety fellow of the author's patient safety fellowship studied orthostatic hypotension in an inpatient psychiatric ward as part of a quality project addressing falls. He found that in a convenience cohort of Caucasian men older than 55 receiving antihypertensive medication, those taking 2 or more antipsychotic medications had a greater than 50% chance of having objective evidence of orthostatic hypotension (Hammond Kwame Adjei, PharmD, 2014, unpublished data). The data correlating hip fracture risk with medication usage in large studies is convincing; 2 representative studies will be reviewed.

Lai and colleagues utilized insurance data to compare a cohort of 2328 elderly patients who had suffered hip fracture and over 9000 controls. The authors correlated the number of medications with the risk of fracture. Nearly 10% of the fracture patients utilized 5 or more medications daily, and the odds ratio for a fall-induced hip fracture occurring in patients using 10 or more medications per day was 8.4 when compared with those using 0 or only 1 medication. Age strongly impacted their study, so that when age and numbers of medications were combined, the risk of a fracture increased 23-fold for patients older than 85 years using 10 or more medications per day when compared with those 65 to 74 years of age using 0 or 1 medication.[7] Kaukonen and colleagues correlated medication use with the risk of suffering a second hip fracture. The authors followed a cohort of 221 patients who had suffered an index hip fracture. Patients were followed for 5 years, with a second fall with fracture occurring in 26 (12%), with a mean interval of 4 years between the fractures. At the time of the original fracture, 36% of patients were taking 5 or more medications; at the time of the second fracture, 68% were taking 5 or more medications. The number of patients taking at least one psychoactive drug rose from 36% to 64%.[8]

Although there is convincing evidence that overmedication increases the risk of falls and fractures, the challenge of polypharmacy remains. The author encounters any number of patients on a weekly basis in his practice who have imbalance or orthostatic hypotension due to overmedication. When advised that their medications may be contributing to their complaints, patients are often reluctant to consider discussing medication reduction with their PCPs, since their anxiolytics often enable them to function.

Selective serotonin reuptake inhibitors (SSRIs) present a conundrum in the management of older adults with depression and balance difficulties. The 2010 AGS/BGS CPG briefly addresses the evidence, which, in contrast to tricyclic antidepressants, is not overwhelming. Mark and colleagues pointed out that older adults who are on antidepressants are also often on more drugs of other classes than patients without depression, confusing the clinical correlation.[9] There is evidence that SSRIs vary in their anticholinergic properties. As such, there may be some value in transitioning patients with balance disorders to a less-impairing SSRI.[10]

EVALUATION OF THE OLDER ADULT WITH A BALANCE DISORDER

The AGS/BGS CPG emphasizes that the evaluation of fall risk in an older adult includes not only a history of falls, but also an objective assessment of balance. The assessment should include an assessment of gait, which the author believes should be performed without the patient aware that gait is being evaluated. The get up and go test, as well as an evaluation of gait speed, may be helpful. Assessment of vision is important, and it is expeditious to evaluate the vestibular-ocular reflex (VOR) at the same time by testing vision with the head stationary and while moving it side to side. Evaluation for orthostatic hypotension should be performed if the history is suggestive. If a standard Romberg test is negative, it can be enhanced by asking the patient to stand on a compliant surface, or to attempt to stand on 1 leg (recognizing that most older individuals cannot perform this task). If there is any history suggestive of BPPV, a Dix Hallpike test should be performed, as BPPV often occurs in concert with balance disorders. Although many otolaryngologists routinely utilize formal vestibular testing such as rotational chair, caloric, and postural testing, the author tends to avoid these in older adults, since they are uncomfortable and rarely influence treatment.

MANAGEMENT

The initial intervention is often modification of the patient's medications. It is not uncommon to encounter patients who have been started on meclizine for BPPV or presbystasis, for which the medication is contraindicated. Inducing the patient to consider discontinuing other antihistamines, anticholinergics, or benzodiazepams is more challenging, and the author is rarely successful in this regard. Advising the patient to monitor his or her own blood pressure and to report to his or her PCP may be efficacious in adjusting antihypertensive medications. Finally, educating PCPs and other nongeriatricians regarding the existence of the Beers criteria may be helpful. The author is continually surprised that many PCPs are unaware of this list and its implications for the management of older adults.

Beyond medication management, vestibular rehabilitation is the most effective management for presbystasis, postlabyrinthitis vestibulopathy, and many other balance disorders. Unfortunately, many older adults with balance dysfunction are inactive. The author often encounters older adults who, because of fear of falls, restrict their unassisted ambulation to just a few meters. Many are reliant on motorized scooters, essentially depriving themselves of the benefit of exercise and balance. Formal vestibular rehabilitation is more than ambulation, but includes many movements that closely resemble dancing. Unfortunately, like any exercise program, having 1 or 2 sessions weekly is suboptimal. Rather, 3 or 4 sessions per week should be the minimum. Fortunately, many age-specific exercise classes focus on just this type of exercise, and provide interaction with peers as an added benefit. There are excellent data supporting the value of Tai Chi and yoga in maintaining balance. For patients who are able, the author recommends joining a dance class. There is evidence supporting effectiveness of the Wii Fit and similar game devices in enhancing balance function. Primary care-directed and -monitored balance rehabilitation exercise programs have been demonstrated to be successful.[11] It is the author's opinion that the widespread dissemination of programs of this nature have the potential to reduce the burden of balance disorders in the geriatric population. Furthermore, one can anticipate that new technology using virtual reality may soon provide additional opportunities for enjoyable and effective balance exercises for the aging population.

SUMMARY

Balance disorders are common, affecting approximately one-third of older adults. Most of these disorders are variants of presbystasis, often aggravated by medications and inactivity. Evaluation should focus on addressing common vestibular disorders, particularly BPPV, and reduction in medications, particularly psychoactive medications. Orthostatic hypotension should be considered in patients with a suggestive history. All patients should be encouraged to participate in a regular balance exercise program, hopefully in a setting that is enjoyable in order to maintain ongoing interest and participation. Geriatricians should take an active role in educating PCPs and other nongeriatricians in the evaluation and management of older adults with balance disorders.

REFERENCES

1. Lin HW, Bhattacharyya N. Balance disorders in the elderly: epidemiology and functional impact. Laryngoscope 2012;122:1858–61.
2. Agrawal Y, Carey JP, Della Santini CC, et al. Disorders of balance and vestibular function in US adults: data from the National Nutrition and Health Examination 2001-2004. Arch Intern Med 2009;169:938–44.
3. Panel on Prevention of Falls in Older Persons, American Geriatrics Society and British Geriatrics Society. Summary of the updated American Geriatrics Society/British Geriatrics Society Clinical Practice Guideline for prevention of falls in older persons. J Am Geriatr Soc 2011;59(1):148–57. Available at: http://www. geriatricscareonline.org/ProductAbstract/updated-american-geriatrics-society british-geriatrics-society-clinical-practice-guideline-for-prevention-of-falls-in-older-persons-and-recommendations/CL014.
4. Furman JM, Raz Y, Whitney SL. Geriatric vestibulopathy assessment and management. Curr Opin Otolaryngol Head Neck Surg 2010;18:386–91.
5. Ciorba A, Hatzopoulos S, Bianchini C, et al. Genetics of presbycusis and presbystasis. Int J Immunopathol Pharmacol 2015;28:29–35.
6. Bhattacharyya N, Gubbels SP, Schwartz SR, et al. Clinical practice guideline: benign paroxysmal positional vertigo (update). Otolaryngol Head Neck Surg 2017;156:S1–47. Available at: http://journals.sagepub.com/doi/abs/10.1177/0194599816689667?url_ver=Z39.88-2003&rfr_id=ori%3Arid%3Acrossref.org&rfr_dat=cr_pub%3Dpubmed&.
7. Lai S, Liao K, Liao C, et al. Polypharmacy correlates with increased risk for hip fractgure in the elderly: a population-based study. Medicine 2010;89:295–9.
8. Kaukonen JP, Luthje P, Nurmi-Luthje I, et al. Second hip fracture and patients medication after the first hip fracture: a follow-up of 221 hip fracture patients in Finland. Arch Gerontol Geriatr 2011;52:185–9.
9. Mark TL, Joish VN, Hay JW, et al. Antidepressant use in geriatric populations: the burden of side effects and interactions and their impact on adherence and costs. Am J Geriatr Psychiatry 2011;19:211–23.
10. Sanchez C, Reines EH, Montgomery SA. A comparative review of escitalopram, paroxetine, and sertraline: are they all alike? Int Clin Psychopharmacol 2014;29:185–96.
11. Yardley L, Donovan-Hall M, Smith SE, et al. Effectiveness of primary care–based vestibular rehabilitation for chronic dizziness. Ann Intern Med 2004;141:598–605.

Geriatric Dysphagia

Ozlem E. Tulunay-Ugur, MD[a],*, David Eibling, MD[b]

KEYWORDS

- Geriatric dysphagia • Dysphagia team • Aspiration pneumonia
- Cricopharyngeal spasm

KEY POINTS

- All geriatric patients should be screened for potential dysphagia. Because swallowing problems can be regarded as a normal part of aging by patients and families, it may not be brought up as a complaint unless the physician makes a specific inquiry.
- The key to diagnosis lies in a detailed and thorough history. Reported symptoms will guide further testing. Similarly, detailed understanding of the current diet will determine the urgency of intervention to improve nutritional intake and prevent complications such as aspiration pneumonia.
- Successful management requires a dysphagia team. Although many surgical treatment options are available, the most important part of successful management is rehabilitation and diet modification.

INTRODUCTION

Among the disorders precipitated by diseases accompanying aging, perhaps that with the most impact on quality of life is dysphagia. This is particularly true in patients who have undergone treatment of tumors of the head and neck, who are often affected with severe dysphagia that worsens with age and is discussed elsewhere in this issue. However, many other ailments of aging, common and uncommon, affect swallowing. The extent of the problem is immense, with 40% of institutionalized older adults having a diagnosis of dysphagia. In some instances, the effect on swallowing leads to death due to aspiration or inanition. The otolaryngologist plays a central role in the management of dysphagia, not only as the treating physician but also as the expert guiding crucial end-of-life decisions. This article focuses on critical knowledge to guide clinical decision-making rather than technical details of workup and surgical procedures.

Disclosures: None.
[a] Department of Otolaryngology–Head and Neck Surgery, University of Arkansas for Medical Sciences, 4301 West Markham Street, Slot 543, Little Rock, AR 72223, USA; [b] Department of Otolaryngology–Head and Neck Surgery, University of Pittsburgh, Eye and Ear Institute, Suite 500, 203 Lothrop Street, Pittsburgh, PA 15213, USA
* Corresponding author.
E-mail address: oetulunayugur@uams.edu

Clin Geriatr Med 34 (2018) 183–189
https://doi.org/10.1016/j.cger.2018.01.007
0749-0690/18/Published by Elsevier Inc.

Normal Swallowing Function

There are numerous texts describing normal and abnormal swallowing function; therefore, this article only reviews the highlights. Normal swallowing is empirically divided into 4 phases, the first 2 of which, the oral preparatory phase and the oral phase (often referred to as the horizontal subsystem), create and move the bolus under voluntary control into position, then triggering the so called vertical subsystem by pressure against the soft palate. The vertical subsystem consists of the involuntary laryngopharyngeal and the esophageal phases, moving the bolus through the pharynx, by the larynx, and through the esophagus into the stomach. Although often addressed as separate functions, in reality all phases are coordinated and often overlap significantly. Failure in any of the phases, such as inability to form a cohesive bolus during mastication, can impair the function of the pharyngeal phase. Although clinical evaluations typically focus on the laryngopharyngeal phase because it is this phase in which the greatest number of coordinated events must occur, impairment often occurs in multiple phases. Airway protection must precede bolus transport, and must be maintained until the bolus has passed in its entirety. Glottic closure during the laryngopharyngeal phase occurs in a different sequence than closure for coughing or speech, and hyolaryngeal elevation not only cantilevers the epiglottis over the glottic opening but also actively distracts the cricoid ring to distract the cricopharyngeal (CP) muscle and open the upper esophageal sphincter (UES). Moving the bolus through the pharynx and UES requires only about 0.7 seconds in normal young individuals but may be prolonged in normal-aged but asymptomatic individuals. Once through the UES into the esophagus, orderly peristaltic waves transport the bolus at a velocity of 2 to 4 cm/s into the distal esophagus, then through the lower esophageal sphincter, requiring less than 10 seconds in normal patients. The upper esophagus, consisting of striated muscle, is under central neural control, as are the pharyngeal muscles; however, the smooth muscle of the distal esophagus is intrinsically innervated, as well as subject to extrinsic control by the vagus.

Normal Swallowing in the Elderly

Swallowing changes, often termed presbyphagia, occur with normal aging. An understanding of swallowing in the normal elderly, as well as knowledge of the range of disorders is needed in planning interventions.

Robbins and colleagues[1] have extensively studied and described swallowing in normal, community-dwelling older adults. In normal subjects, changes accompanying aging are minimal and are unaccompanied by symptoms, thereby escaping detection except in focused investigations. Some of these changes are listed in **Box 1**. The most

---

Box 1
Characteristics of presbyphagia

Differences in swallowing function in normal-aged individuals

1. Slowing of pressure rise during pharyngeal swallowing

2. Reduced maximum isometric tongue pressure

3. Persistent cricopharyngeal bar on barium studies

4. Persistent residue following swallow

5. Increased likelihood of nonpathologic penetration

6. Various forms of esophageal dysmotility

7. Slowing of esophageal transit time

salient of these changes are slowing of swallowing pressure rise (although ultimate pressures are unchanged from younger individuals), an increased presence of residue following swallowing, and the presence of a persistent CP bar on barium studies. Because these changes are usually asymptomatic, their presence in symptomatic patients may be confusing and lead to an inaccurate diagnosis. It has been hypothesized that the observed slowing is due to the delay in recruiting additional motor units to achieve the required pressures.[2]

Although normal swallowing pressures are measured in the elderly, maximum isometric tongue pressures decrease linearly with aging. This finding suggests that the elderly are using a greater percentage of their tongue strength reserve to maintain normal pressures during swallowing. Moreover, elderly patients may use multiple lingual movement gestures to achieve sufficient pressures. These studies collaborate the observation that older adults eat more slowly, and rarely bolt their food.[2,3] It seems likely that normal adults alter their eating habits to accommodate to these changes. These findings also suggest a mechanism whereby seemingly unrelated illnesses can lead to swallowing morbidity merely as a result of depleting functional reserve. As Robbins and colleagues[1] point out, these perturbations set up the elderly to cross over from a healthy older swallower to a person with dysphagia.

Esophageal motility disorders are so common in the elderly that they should probably be considered a normal variant. In a study of 24 asymptomatic community-dwelling older adults, more than half had objective evidence of dysmotility, including stasis (residual material following primary wave) in 96% and intraesophageal reflux (retrograde movement of bolus before passing the lower esophageal sphincter) in 60%. Findings were substantially more common in older men.[4] These findings indicate that attributing symptoms to radiographic findings may not be appropriate unless the radiologist is familiar with the normal range of findings in the geriatric population.

Evaluation of Swallowing in the Elderly

Knowledge that the elderly are at risk for dysphagia-associated morbidity has driven health care institutions to focus attention on identifying, quantifying, and managing dysphagia in vulnerable populations with the goal of preventing aspiration-related pulmonary disease, as well as malnutrition. To this end, most organizations who care for the elderly or patients with chronic illnesses have well-developed procedures, typically overseen by a speech-language pathologist (SLP)-directed dysphagia team. The value of these teams cannot be overemphasized and physicians who manage vulnerable patients, such as the elderly, should make an effort to become familiar with the team in their facility, as well as their operational strategies and procedures.

Stroke patients are at significant risk for dysphagia-related comorbidities, which may lead to mortality; hence, prospective screening of these patients has been guideline-driven since 2005.[5] Some facilities, such as Veteran Affairs hospitals, use a nurse-driven standard screening process for all at-risk patients to identify patients that need further workup by SLP. Other centers are staffed adequately to enable SLP screening of all at-risk patients at admission, whereas in others evaluation will occur only on specific consultation by the treating team. Typically, dysphagia evaluation in the outpatient arena is sporadic at best, except in formal protocoled clinics such as survivor clinics and this is discussed elsewhere in this issue.

Unfortunately, bedside evaluation of many patients with neurologic disease is impaired by reduced sensation. It is self-evident that the presence of a gag reflex does not correlate with safe swallowing. As a result of sensory impairment, as many as 50% of these patients may demonstrate silent aspiration, meaning that aspiration does not trigger a cough. Identification of specific aspects of swallowing function, particularly silent aspiration, is best demonstrated by either radiographic contrast studies, the so-called modified barium swallow (MBS) in most institutions, or direct vision of the pharynx, the fiberoptic (or flexible) endoscopic evaluation of swallowing (FEES). A full discussion of these techniques is beyond the intent of this article and the reader is referred to the many excellent texts on the topic. Regardless, the physician managing the patient should make every effort to review either the recorded MBS or the FEES examination of their patients with dysphagia to help guide decision-making.

Dysphagia due to Polypharmacy

Essentially all practitioners are familiar with the concepts of dysphagia associated with obstructive lesions or neurogenic disorders such as stroke, progressive neurodegenerative diseases, and so forth. However, the role of medications in inducing or aggravating dysphagia in the elderly is less appreciated and deserves some discussion. Dysphagia due to medications can be divided into 2 major categories: those medications that reduce the amount or increase the viscosity of saliva, and centrally acting sedatives that impair the complex neurologic-driven interplay of the multiple components of swallowing. Among the former, the most common are diuretics and anticholinergic medications, both of which are commonly encountered on medication lists of elderly patients. Not only does the presence of adherent mucus impair swallowing but also the loss of the normal rinsing effect of saliva in the esophagus may contribute to esophagitis. The role of selective serotonin reuptake inhibitors is controversial in the geriatric literature, and the anticholinergic effect may vary widely among the different formulations.

Among the common sedatives are benzodiazepines and antihistamines, again frequently encountered on review of medication lists. The effect of the drying agents is easily seen on fiberoptic examination, and the effect of the sedatives can be visualized on MBS or FEES. Many of these medications are listed in the Beers criteria as being potentially inappropriate for older adults. Joint management of geriatric patients with geriatricians is significantly helpful in the management of patients with swallowing disorders.[6]

Treatment

The management strategies can be divided into conservative through the use of swallowing therapy and nutritional modifications, and surgical. In a review of all patients presenting to a tertiary care center with dysphagia who suffered from no neurologic disorders or head and neck cancer, the authors noted that about 30% of the patients required a surgical intervention, whereas 60% needed diet modification, and another 22% needed swallowing therapy.[7] Hence, the role of a team approach with SLPs, nutritionists, and occupational therapists in the forefront of the management of the elderly patients with dysphagia cannot be overemphasized.

There continues to be no consensus on how to select patients requiring surgical intervention. This remains true for the 2 primarily surgical disorders of the elderly, which are CP muscle dysfunction and Zenker diverticulum. CP dysfunction, which can lead to solid food dysphagia, aspiration, weight loss, and reduced quality of life, can result from anatomic, neuromuscular, iatrogenic, inflammatory, neoplastic, or idiopathic cause.[8] Without well-established guidelines, management depends on surgeon preferences and background. The traditional surgical treatment of CP spasm has been myotomy through a transcervical approach. Endoscopic myotomy was introduced by Halvorson and Kuhn[9] using the potassium-titanyl-phosphate laser (KTP) in the early 1990s. The carbon dioxide (CO_2) laser later replaced the KTP due to better coagulative abilities. The technique has been comprehensively described by Pitman and Weissbrod[10] in their 2009 paper detailing the procedure. As long as the buccopharyngeal pharyngeal fascia is preserved and the retropharyngeal space left undisturbed, endoscopic myotomy has been shown to be a safe and effective procedure in most patients.[11] Regrettably, the fear of mediastinitis continues to discourage many otolaryngologists from performing CO_2 laser myotomy. In a systematic review that evaluated the most commonly used techniques in the treatment of CP spasm, comparing endoscopic versus open myotomy, botulinum toxin injections, and dilatation outcomes and complications, it was demonstrated that best functional outcomes were achieved with endoscopic myotomy. Moreover, when complication rates were compared, logistic regression analysis showed a significant increase in the odds of complication with the open procedure.[12] Botulinum toxin injections into the CP muscle, first described by Blitzer and Brin[13] in 1993, can be performed under direct visualization and general anesthesia or in the office with electromyographic guidance. There is no agreement on the dose needed and it ranges from 10 U to 100 U in the literature.[14] Complications may arise from the injection or diffusion of the toxin into the inferior constrictor muscles, which can lead to worsening dysphagia, aspiration, and need for percutaneous endoscopic gastrostomy (PEG) tube placement; or into the posterior cricoarytenoid muscles, which can lead to respiratory compromise if both sides are affected. Mortality has been reported related to botulinum toxin injection, likely related to aspiration due to the injection of the inferior constrictors.[15] Hence, patient selection requires diligence and careful discussion of expected outcomes. Treatment should be offered to patients with dysfunctional CP muscle, who are symptomatic with additional clinical findings, such as flexible laryngoscopic examination showing pooling in the pyriform sinuses and an MBS demonstrating a CP bar. Although preferred, intact pharyngeal contraction is not a prerequisite for surgical management, as shown by Kos and colleagues.[16] In their series, 71% of subjects with normal constriction showed improvement, and 79% of subjects with reduced activity and 71% with absent activity also showed improvement in swallowing. As in any surgery on the elderly, risks of general anesthesia should be weighed; frailty and diminished functional reserve can lead to poor perioperative outcomes. It has been demonstrated that geriatric consultation improves outcomes in older patients, and can aid in decision-making.[17,18]

Similar to CP dysfunction, well-established guidelines are lacking in the management of Zenker diverticulum, and management and chosen surgical technique heavily rely on surgeon comfort. Various techniques have been described, and endoscopic techniques are preferred by most surgeons due to shorter surgical times, shorter hospital stay, earlier return to normal diet, and improved complication rates.[19,20] A 2015 systematic review by Verdonck and Morton[21] assessed treatment modalities, comparing open versus endoscopic techniques, and endoscopic stapling versus laser-assisted diverticulotomy. They reported failure of open and endoscopic approaches to be 4.2% and 18.4%, respectively, with corresponding complication rates of 11% and 7%. Within endoscopic techniques, failure rates were 18.9% for stapler diverticulotomy and 21.7% for laser diverticulotomy. Corresponding complication rates were 4.3% and 7.9%. Flexible endoscopic techniques had a higher failure (29%) and overall complication rate (14.3%). Most reported complications for transcervical techniques were related to the recurrent nerve (3.4%) and salivary fistula formation (3.7%), whereas in the endoscopic group emphysema (3.0%) and mediastinitis (1.2%) were the most common complications. Operation-related deaths were infrequent in both groups but more frequent with the open approach (0.9 vs 0.4%). They concluded open approaches had more success but more complications than endoscopic techniques, and recommended an open approach in younger patients, as well in patients with unfavorable anatomic conditions for endoscopic exposure. Flexible endoscopic techniques were noted to provide a suitable option for patients who cannot tolerate general anesthesia. The results from Agalato and colleagues[22] were contrary to this and they reported improved outcomes with open procedures. In their series of 97 subjects, the complication rates were less in the endoscopic group with 15% versus 25% in the open procedure group, but with 1 mortality in the endoscopic group. Symptom recurrence was significantly higher in the endoscopic group (26% vs 7%) and multiple procedures were required in this group. Their conclusion was that endoscopic approaches did not have a significant advantage over open techniques. Barton and colleagues[23] compared laser-assisted with stapler-assisted diverticulotomy and demonstrated comparable success and complication rates. The addition of the laser-assisted approach to the surgical armamentarium increased the successful completion rates of endoscopic procedures because fewer surgical procedures were aborted due to exposure problems or size criteria. Recently, there is increased reporting of flexible endoscopic myotomy for the management of Zenker diverticulum, with most of the literature coming from European gastroenterologists.[24,25] Further clinical experience is needed to understand the value of this technique.

SUMMARY

Dysphagia in the elderly may be associated with morbidity and potentially even mortality. As such, it requires a thorough, diligent evaluation and team approach. Due to the complex nature of swallowing, increased comorbidities in older adults, and the dismissal of many problems in this patient population as normal aging, the diagnosis and management of clinically significant dysphagia may be delayed. This not only leads to a substantial decrease in quality of life but also places the patient at risk for malnutrition, aspiration, and death. A good understanding of both the swallowing disorders in this age group and the available management options is required to optimize care in this vulnerable population.

REFERENCES

1. Robbins JA, Connor, Barczi. Effects of aging on swallowing. In: Calhoun, Eibling, editors. Geriatric otolaryngology. New York: 2006.
2. Robins J, Levine R, Wood J, et al. Age effects on lingual pressure generation as a risk factor for dysphagia. J Gerontol A Biol Sci Med Sci 1995;50:M257–62.
3. Nicosia MA, Hind JA, Roecker EB, et al. Age effects on the temporal evolution of isometric and swallowing pressure. J Gerontol A Biol Sci Med Sci 2000;55: M634–40.
4. Jou J, Radowsky J, Gangnon R, et al. Esophageal clearance patterns in normal older adults as documented with videofluoroscopic esophagram. Gastroenterol Res Pract 2009;2009:965062.
5. Bates B, Choi JY, Duncan PW, et al. Veterans affairs/Department of defense clinical practice guideline for the management of adult stroke rehabilitation care: executive summary. Stroke 2005;36:2049–56.
6. Gallagher L, Naidoo P. Prescription drugs and their effects on swallowing. Dysphagia 2009;24:159–66.
7. Kocdor P, Siegel ER, Giese R, et al. Characteristics of dysphagia in older patients evaluated at a tertiary center. Laryngoscope 2015;125:400–5.
8. Dauer E, Salassa J, Luga L, et al. Endoscopic laser vs open approach for cricopharyngeal myotomy. Otolaryngol Head Neck Surg 2006;134:830–5.

9. Halvorson DJ, Kuhn FA. Transmucosal cricopharyngeal myotomy with the potassium-titanyl-phosphate laser in the treatment of cricopharyngeal dysmotility. Ann Otol Rhinol Laryngol 1994;103:173–7.
10. Pitman M, Weissbrod P. Endoscopic CO2 laser cricopharyngeal myotomy. Laryngoscope 2009;119:45–53.
11. Chang CWD, Liou SS, Netterville JL. Anatomic study of laser-assisted endoscopic cricopharyngeus myotomy. Ann Otol Rhinol Laryngol 2005;114:897–901.
12. Kocdor P, Siegel ER, Tulunay-Ugur OE. Cricopharyngeal dysfunction: a systematic review comparing outcomes of dilatation, botulinum toxin injection, and myotomy. Laryngoscope 2016;126:135–41.
13. Blitzer A, Brin MF. Use of botulinum toxin for diagnosis and management of cricopharyngeal achalasia. Otolaryngol Head Neck Surg 1997;116:328–30.
14. Kim DY, Park CI, Ohn SH, et al. Botulinum toxin type A for post-stroke cricopharyngeal muscle dysfunction. Arch Phys Med Rehabil 2006;87:1346–51.
15. Bammer T, Salassa JR, Klingler PJ. Comparison of methods for determining cricopharyngeal intra-bolus pressure in normal patients as possible indicator for cricopharyngeal myotomy. Otolaryngol Head Neck Surg 2002;127:299–308.
16. Kos MP, David EF, Klinkenberg-Knol EC, et al. Long-term results of external upper esophageal sphincter myotomy for oropharyngeal dysphagia. Dysphagia 2010; 25:169–76.
17. Shuman AG, Korc-Grodzicki B, Shklar V, et al. A new care paradigm in geriatric head and neck surgical oncology. J Surg Oncol 2013;108:187–91.
18. Wong CL, Al Atia R, McFarlan A, et al. Sustainability of a proactive geriatric trauma consultation service. Can J Surg 2017;60:14–8.
19. Richtsmeier WJ. Endoscopic management of Zenker diverticulum: the staple assisted approach. Am J Med 2003;115:175S–8S.
20. Leong SC, Wilkie MD, Webb CJ. Endoscopic stapling of Zenker's diverticulum: establishing national baselines for auditing clinical outcomes in the United Kingdom. Eur Arch Otorhinolaryngol 2012;269:1877–84.
21. Verdonck J, Morton RP. Systematic review on treatment of Zenker's diverticulum. Eur Arch Otorhinolaryngol 2015;272:3095–107.
22. Agalato E, Jose J, England RJ. Is pharyngeal pouch stapling superior to open pharyngeal pouch repair? An analysis of a single institution's series. J Laryngol Otol 2016;130:873–7.
23. Barton MD, Detwiller KY, Palmer AD, et al. The safety and efficacy of endoscopic Zenker's diverticulotomy: A cohort study. Laryngoscope 2016;126:2705–10.
24. Dişibeyaz S, Kuzu UB, Parlak E, et al. Endoscopic treatment of the Zenker diverticulum with flexible endoscopic myotomy: a single tertiary center experience. Surg Laparosc Endosc Percutan Tech 2017;27(6):e136–40.
25. Wilmsen J, Baumbach R, Stüker D, et al. New flexible endoscopic controlled stapler technique for the treatment of Zenker's diverticulum: a case series. World J Gastroenterol 2017;23(17):3084–91.

Voice Disorders in the Elderly

Karen M. Kost, MD, FRCSC[a],*, Robert T. Sataloff, MD, DMA[b]

KEYWORDS

- Presbyphonia • Vocal atrophy • Physiology of aging voice • Acoustics of aging voice
- Quality of life • Voice therapy • Vocal exercise • Singing

KEY POINTS

- Dysphonia in the elderly is a common and likely underreported symptom.
- There are key anatomic and physiologic changes contributing to the aging voice.
- Singing largely prevents or mitigates changes associated with the aging voice.
- Vocal exercises are of proven benefit in presbyphonia
- Surgical options such as vocal fold injection augmentation and thyroplasty may offer additional improvement.

INTRODUCTION

As the number of individuals aged 65 and older increases, it is not surprising to note an increase in the number of older patients seeking consultations for dysphonia. The reported incidence of vocal complaints in the geriatric population is somewhere between 12% and 35%.[1,2] In developed countries, older individuals comprise an increasing proportion of the workforce. Twenty to 35% of geriatric patients (Kost K, Yammine N. Dysphonia in the elderly: findings from the McGill Voice Laboratory; unpublished data, 2012)[3] use their voices for work, suggesting that vocal health is a high priority within this subgroup of older patients. In all geriatric patients, dysphonia negatively impacts quality of life. Often, it also significantly impairs the ability to communicate effectively with hearing-impaired spouses, family, and friends. Indeed, dysphonia

Modified in part from: Sataloff RT, Johns MM, Kost KM. *Geriatric otolaryngology.* New York (NY): Thieme Publishing, Inc; 2015; with permission; and Sataloff RT. *Professional voice: the science and art of clinical care, third edition.* San Diego (CA): Plural Publishing, Inc; 2005; with permission.
Disclosures: None.
[a] Department of Otolaryngology-Head and Neck Surgery, McGill University Health Centre, Room DS1-3310, 1001 Decarie Bouleard, Montreal, Quebec H4A 3J1, Canada; [b] Department of Otolaryngology–Head and Neck Surgery, Drexel University College of Medicine, Philadelphia, PA, USA
* Corresponding author.
E-mail address: kmkost@yahoo.com

and hearing loss frequently coexist in the elderly; those with hearing loss are more likely to have dysphonia than their counterparts without hearing loss.[4] Consequently, dysphonic seniors may suffer from social isolation, anxiety, and depression, indicating a need to address both dysphonia and hearing loss when treating these patients.[2,5]

Presbyphonia should not be diagnosed until all other possibilities have been considered and eliminated. It may also coexist with other vocal diagnoses, including benign vocal fold lesions (polyps, nodules, cysts, papillomas), chronic inflammatory laryngitis (reflux-related conditions, autoimmune disorders, medication-induced conditions), acute inflammatory laryngitis (viral, fungal, and bacterial), muscle tension disorders, neurologic disorders (essential tremor, Parkinson's, poststroke, spasmodic dysphonia, amyotrophic lateral sclerosis), vocal malignancies, vocal fold immobility (from mechanical or neurologic causes), and vocal fold paresis of the superior or recurrent laryngeal nerve. Vocal fold atrophy is unusual in younger patients except in the setting of muscle wasting diseases, paresis and paralysis, or extreme weight loss. Despite the high prevalence of dysphonia in the elderly, there are relatively few published studies on the subject. This may be because of the complexity of the subject; the severity of dysphonia in the geriatric patient is a function of not only the primary vocal diagnosis, but also several other factors including the functional status of the patient, coexisting morbidities, pulmonary reserve, medications, and cognitive function.

In a retrospective review of 175 elderly patients seen in a tertiary care laryngology practice in Philadelphia, the most common complaints were hoarseness in 71%, inability to project the voice or decreased volume in 45%, excessive throat clearing and phlegm in 43%, vocal fatigue in 37%, cough in 23%, and breathiness in 22%.[6] Less common complaints included raspiness, pitch breaks, loss of range, globus sensation, tremor, and dysphagia. Many patients had more than 1 complaint. The most commonly identified diagnoses, which frequently coexisted with other conditions such as presbylarynx, included laryngopharyngeal reflux, muscle tension dysphonia, paresis (diagnosed clinically and with electromyography in many cases), vocal fold mass, glottic insufficiency, and varicosities and ectasias. As a result of their dysphonia, more than 50% of patients in this study reported a significant impairment in their quality of life, with potentially serious psychosocial implications.[6]

ANATOMY AND PHYSIOLOGY

With advancing age, the respiratory system undergoes marked anatomic and physiologic changes, with a net decrease or undermining of the power source of the voice.[7–11] The larynx itself also undergoes extensive anatomic and physiologic change during adulthood,[12] as summarized in previous literature.[13] Changes in the larynx from young adulthood to old age are generally more extensive in men than in women, with the possible exception of muscle atrophy, about which there is little information on gender differences.[12] The nature of age-related changes in the epithelium of the vocal folds has been in dispute. Several investigators report thickening; others have found no evidence of change with aging.

Microscopic changes noted in the superficial layer of the lamina propria have been documented, including thickening or edema of the superficial layer, degeneration or atrophy of elastic fibers, and decreases in the number of myofibrils.[14,15] Histologic examination of aged human vocal folds has shown a decrease in the total number of cells, a decrease in the intracellular organelles responsible for protein synthesis, and reduced production of extracellular matrix from these cells. The overall result is that the superficial layer of the lamina propria increases in thickness and is more edematous in both men and women, with a change in viscoelastic properties.[16,17] Changes within the cricoarytenoid joint include surface irregularities and disorganization of collagen fibers.[18] Laryngeal cartilages stiffen with progressive calcification and/ or ossification.[19–21]

A great deal of work, summarized by Thomas and colleagues,[22] has revealed changes in the musculature of the aging larynx, which contribute significantly to presbyphonia. A number of skeletal muscle changes are known to occur with aging. Although many of these also apply to the thyroarytenoid (TA) muscle, there are also notable differences. Sarcopenia refers to the loss in muscle mass, strength, and quality often observed with aging. Because the loss in muscle mass is gradual, there is little noticeable loss in function, until the loss extends beyond threshold levels. At this point, functional abilities decrease noticeably. Sarcopenia is likely the result of metabolic, neurologic, hormonal, and environmental factors.

The TA muscle extends from the thyroid cartilage anteriorly to the vocal process and fovea oblonga of the arytenoid cartilage.[22] It is often thought of as being made up of a medial vocalis and more laterally positioned thyromuscularis (**Fig. 1**). The latter probably plays a role in the rapid shortening of the vocal fold, whereas the vocalis is likely involved in fine-tuning the tension along the vocal fold edge, and in providing lateral resistance during vocal fold contact. Contraction of the TA muscle results in thickening and stiffening of the vocal fold, and a corresponding loosening of the lamina propria. Compared with limb skeletal muscle, the TA muscle differs in several ways, including fiber size, contractile protein profiles, mitochondrial content, and aging patterns. Similar differences also have been found in other laryngeal muscles.

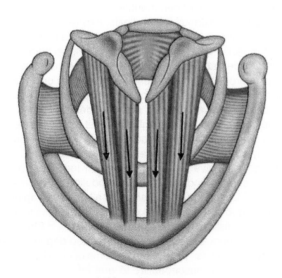

Action of vocalis
(thyroarytenoid) muscles

Fig. 1. The thyroarytenoid muscle which consists of the medially positioned vocalis and the more laterally positioned thyromuscularis. (*From* Sataloff RT, Chowdhury F, Portnoy JE, et al. Anatomy and physiology of the voice: a brief overview. In: Sataloff RT, Chowdhury F, Portnoy JE, et al, editors. Surgical techniques in otolaryngology – head and neck surgery: laryngeal surgery. New Delhi, India: Jaypee Brothers Medical Publishers; 2014. p. 11; with permission.)

The TA muscle in humans contains types I, IIX, and IIA fibers, as well as fibers.[22] Furthermore, it has been suggested that the fast and slow fibers are arranged along a gradient, with the medial aspect composed of slow fibers and the lateral aspect composed of fast fibers. This unique composition results in a rapidly contracting, fatigue-resistant muscle that is well-suited for the role of the TA muscle as a muscle of respiration, airway protection, and voice production, is unusual compared with limb skeletal muscle. Increased levels of mitochondria have been noted in the posterior cricoarytenoid, cricothyroid, and TA muscles compared with limb skeletal muscle. This feature may increase resistance to fatigue and facilitate the continuous action required by these muscles for respiration. The TA muscle is richly innervated by the recurrent laryngeal and superior laryngeal branches of the vagus nerve. Motor units are small, with each motor neuron innervating only a few fibers. Laryngeal sensory information is received through mechanoreceptors, chemoreceptors, taste buds, and free nerve endings.

Although the loss of muscle mass with aging in the human TA muscle was identified first in 1941, and confirmed in subsequent studies, patterns of fiber loss have not been defined clearly.[22] In older rats, a reduction in force, speed, and endurance has been identified. Changes in the innervation of the TA muscle with age also have been noted. Although there seems to be no net loss of myelinated or unmyelinated fibers with age, there is an increase in myelin-abnormal and myelin-thinning fibers, suggesting an active process of degeneration and regeneration. In the superior laryngeal nerve, there is a decrease in the size and number of myelinated fibers, which correlates with the documented decrease in laryngeal sensitivity with age. Metabolic changes have been noted also in the aging TA muscle. Mitochondrial DNA mutations consisting of the 4977-base pair deletion have been identified, and these are thought to result in the increased production of injurious free radicals. Expression of this mutation seems to increase with age, producing dysfunctional mitochondria that may affect contractile properties of the TA muscle negatively. In addition, laryngeal blood flow decreases by approximately 50% in older rats, with a possible reduction in oxygen, and an accumulation of cellular waste products. The influence of hormones on vocal maturation, and in senescence, is recognized widely, and appreciated clinically. The mechanism of action of these hormones, however, remains poorly understood.

Marked anatomic changes in the supraglottic vocal tract have been reported from young adulthood to old age. Changes in facial muscles include decreased elasticity, reduced blood supply, atrophy, and collagen fiber breakdown.[23,24] The temporomandibular joints undergo extensive changes with aging including thinning of articular discs, reduced blood supply, and regressive remodeling of the mandibular condyle and glenoid fossa.[25–30] Dental structures also are altered with aging, although tooth loss itself is not an inevitable consequence of aging.[31] Changes in the tongue epithelium include thinning and fissuring of the tongue surface.[32,33] Pharyngeal and palatal muscles also have been reported to undergo age-related degenerative changes.[34–36]

The loss of salivary function can produce symptoms of oral dryness, dysphagia, and oral discomfort in the elderly; susceptibility to oral infection also is reported to increase.[37] The elderly experience significant decreases in tongue strength, and lingual pressure reserves during swallowing, although maximum tongue pressures during swallow events remain stable into old age.[38,39]

ACOUSTIC CHANGES IN THE AGING VOICE

Mueller opined that, "The voice is a mirror of personality and senescence may cloud that image."[40] The aging voice is associated with a change in vocal quality that may be perceived as reduced volume, increased breathiness, a change in pitch, decreased endurance, and reduced vocal range. When listening to speech samples, listeners are reasonably accurate in distinguishing between young, middle, and older age groups. Older voices often are associated with a loss of range and described with undesirable adjectives such as hoarse, raspy, breathy, unsteady, tremulous, and shaky. The elderly are a heterogeneous group, and many of these characteristics are not solely the result of aging, but rather from poor physical conditioning that results in weak respiratory and abdominal muscles and, ultimately, inadequate vocal support. Numerous studies have shown that listeners can generally differentiate between young and old speakers. Aging affects vocal pitch, loudness, and quality, although the effects are highly variable across the aging population.[41]

Speaking fundamental frequency changes with age, although the pattern of change differs for men and women. In men, the fundamental frequency of speaking decreases through about the fifth decade and then increases, perhaps owing to vocal fold muscle atrophy or hormonal changes. In women, speaking fundamental frequency remains fairly constant or decreases slightly until menopause, after which additional decreasing of the fundamental frequency occurs. Interestingly, these changes are less prominent in professional singers who tend to maintain fairly stable fundamental frequency levels throughout adulthood.[42,43] Speech intensity also changes with age, with both genders experiencing a decrease in maximum intensity levels with advancing age.[44,45] In addition, older women cannot phonate as softly as young women, resulting in an increased minimum intensity level.[45]

Although there is variability in vocal intensity with age, most studies[46] agree that in the elderly, vocal intensity of speech and the ability to modulate it are reduced. Notably, these changes are much less apparent in elderly singers compared with nonsingers, supporting a role for vocal exercise.

Jitter and shimmer are higher in the elderly when compared with younger people and have been associated with a higher Voice Handicap Index scores.[6] Both of these characteristics are related to perceptual qualities of harshness and roughness, which have been identified as characteristics of old voices. Singers, as well as other healthy, physically fit older individuals display less jitter and shimmer and sound younger compared with their counterparts in poor health.

Examination of patients with an old voice using strobovideolaryngoscopy may reveal changes associated with vocal atrophy including variable degrees of bowing, noted as a concavity of the medial edge of the vocal fold during both adduction and abduction, prominent vocal processes, a spindle-shaped glottic chink, and a reduction in amplitude of the mucosal wave[47,48] (**Figs. 2** and **3**).

Although some age-related alterations cannot be avoided in specific individuals, not all of them are manifestations of irreversible deterioration. In fact, as our understanding of the aging process improves, it is becoming more and more apparent that many of these changes can be forestalled or even corrected. As physicians and teachers, we need to look closer before concluding, "I can't help your voice; you're just getting older."

MEDICAL INTERVENTION

Systematically attacking the aging process in other areas of the body is important. The bodily changes characteristic of aging are not unique. In many ways, they are similar to those seen in disuse, such as prolonged bed rest or immobilization. In skeletal muscle of the limbs, muscle disuse and inactivity leads to atrophy, which becomes increasingly difficult to reverse with advancing age. Conversely, high levels of activity,

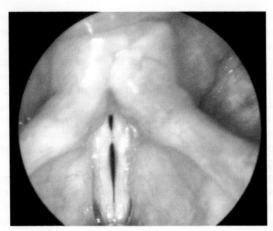

Fig. 2. Photo adducted vocal folds demonstrating typical changes associated with the aging voice. Note the bowed vocal folds, spindle-shaped glottis gap, and prominent vocal processes, all associated with vocal fold atrophy.

including exercise programs, positively affect both the structure and function of muscle. Resistance training increases muscle mass and strength, whereas endurance training increases mitochondrial density and may help to preserve normal muscle morphology. At a cellular level, exercise positively affects hormonal levels, neuronal input, and enzymatic as well as antioxidant activity. This finding suggests that decline is not inevitable, and can be forestalled by optimizing health and physical conditioning. Appropriate exercise not only helps to maintain muscle function and coordination, but also positively impacts the cardiovascular system, nervous system, and especially the respiratory system. Respiratory function, which powers the voice, normally decreases

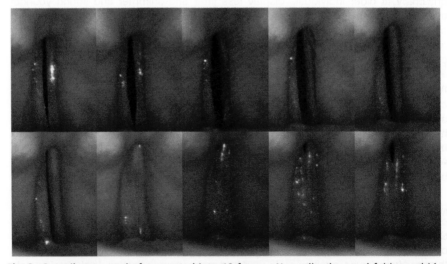

Fig. 3. One vibratory cycle fragmented into 10 frames. Normally, the vocal folds would be adducted in 5 of the frames. Note the presence of a glottis gap in 6 of the 10 frames, as typically seen if vocal atrophy.

with advancing age. In particular, residual lung volume increases, with a consequent decrease in vital capacity, further underlining the importance of optimum respiratory conditioning and good abdominal support. Proper nutrition and weight control also are important. A well-balanced, nutritionally sound diet along with maintaining an optimal weight contributes to a higher quality voice. Oral health includes adequate salivary quality and flow, good dental hygiene, and treatment of any mucosal disorders. Many medications are associated with undesirable effects such as cough, drying effects, and altered cognition, all of which may impact voice negatively. Whenever possible, such medications should be minimized or changed. Reflux should be identified and treated.

For professional singers, audiences have established a certain level of performance that is acceptable. Through optimization of training, physical conditioning, exercise, medication, and other medical conditions, older singers may maximize potential performance level, enabling professionally acceptable performances to be maintained for many decades. Regular vocal technical training can often eliminate the tremolo ("wobble") and improve agility, accuracy, and endurance in the older speaker or singer just as it can in the beginner. For this reason, in treating age-related dysphonia, traditional voice therapy, singing training, acting voice techniques, and aerobic conditioning are often combined to improve neuromuscular performance. It is untrue, indeed unfair, to presume the undesirable characteristics of an older voice are a necessary part of aging. For most patients, rehabilitation restores acceptable voice function and eliminates most of the acoustic information perceived as old. When therapy and medical management alone fail to result in a satisfactory voice, laryngeal surgery may be beneficial.

PSYCHOLOGY AND INTELLECT

Other age-related medical changes also may be significant to vocal function in some people. Clinical observation and decline in cognitive function documented by neuropsychological batteries over time are commonly used to make presumptive diagnoses of Alzheimer's and multiinfarct dementia. Alterations in cognition, especially memory, and changes in personality secondary to mood disorders and delusionality may impair a person's ability to concentrate, consistently perform vocal tasks, and cooperate optimally with voice rehabilitation.

ENDOCRINE SYSTEM

As female singers approach menopause, estrogen deprivation causes substantial changes in the mucous membranes that line the vocal tract, the muscles, and other structures throughout the body, which are frequently reflected in the voice. Although hormone replacement therapy may be helpful, it must be administered with caution and with expert advice because of potential associated risks of increased malignancy. Preparations containing androgens should be avoided in women whenever possible because they can cause masculinization of the voice.

Thyroid disease in the elderly deserves special mention. Both hyperthyroidism and hypothyroidism may be challenging to diagnose in the elderly. Hypothyroidism, for example, frequently does not display "typical" features. Symptoms such as mental slowing, loss of energy, neurotic behavior, hearing loss, weight gain, musculoskeletal discomfort, dry skin, and changes in facial appearance may mistakenly be attributed to age. Alterations in thyroid function frequently produce substantial changes in vocal quality including loss of range, efficiency, and muffling of the voice, all of which resolve with treatment.

HEAD AND NECK

Hearing loss is extremely important in older voice patients. Physicians should determine not only the hearing status of their older voice patients, but also whether they have pitch distortion (diplacusis) and loudness distortion (recruitment).[49] These conditions affect vocal performance, and they may require modifications in rehabilitation strategies. Oral cavity changes associated with aging may be particularly troublesome to singers. Loss of dentition may alter occlusion and articulation, causing especially disturbing problems for professional voice users and wind instrumentalists. These difficulties may be avoided to some extent by having impressions made while dentition is still normal. Dentures that are more similar to the person's natural teeth can then be fashioned. Although salivary glands lose up to about 30% of their parenchymal tissue over a lifetime, salivary secretion remains adequate in most healthy, nonmedicated people throughout life. However, changes in the oral mucosa are similar to those occurring in the skin (thinning and dehydration). They render oral mucosa in the elderly more susceptible to injury, and the sensation of xerostomia may be especially disturbing to singers and other professional voice users. Oral cancers also comprise about 5% of all malignancies, and 95% of oral cancers occur in people over 40 years of age. Cancers in the head and neck may result in profound voice dysfunction.

OTHER CONDITIONS

Many other factors also must be taken into account in the diagnosis and treatment of elderly voice patients. These factors include coronary artery disease, cerebrovascular disease, hypertension, obesity, stroke, diabetes, cancer, diet, osteoporosis, hearing loss, vision loss, swallowing dysfunction, anemia, arthritis, neurologic dysfunction including tremor, incontinence, gastrointestinal disorders, memory and concentration ability, and other conditions. All of these conditions may have adverse effects on the voice either through action directly on the larynx or through impairment of the voice-producing mechanism at another anatomic site that affects, for example, the power source or resonators. Some of these maladies have a major impact on ability to respond to and carry over voice retraining and must be considered when planning therapy for elderly patients.

VOICE THERAPY

Expert voice therapy for presbyphonia is very rewarding, and is best provided by a team, consisting of a physician, speech–language pathologist, singing voice specialist, and frequently an acting voice specialist.[50] In addition to voice therapy, a medically supervised aerobic conditioning program should be considered to restore the power source of the voice, which is essential for both speaking and singing.

The Impact of Vocal Exercise

Voice exercise programs such as Vocal Function Exercises, and Resonant Voice Therapy have been shown to positively affect laryngeal function and voice. Although direct evidence of the effects on TA muscle structure and morphology is lacking, the well-demonstrated benefits of vocal exercise strongly suggest a beneficial effect on the laryngeal musculature. In a study by Gorman and colleagues,[51] 19 elderly men with a diagnosis of presbylarynx were enrolled in a 12-week program of vocal function exercises. At the end of the program, participants demonstrated improved glottic closure, decrease in breathiness, an increase in subglottic pressure, and significantly increased maximum phonation time from 22 to 37 seconds. There is no question that age-related dysphonia impacts quality of life as measured by the validated Voice-Related Quality of Life (VRQOL) survey, a 10-item self-rated questionnaire. Berg and colleagues[52] reported significant improvement in VRQOL scores in 19 elderly patients with dysphonia undergoing voice therapy compared with the 6 controls who chose no treatment. Interestingly, patients who were more compliant with voice therapy had even greater improvements in VRQOLs than those who were less compliant. Although voice therapy is noninvasive, it does require a commitment of time, effort, and resources from elderly patients with age-related dysphonia. Reasonably good cognition is necessary for successful voice therapy.

In the presence of good physical health, technically good singing, which is symbiotic with physical and voice therapy, reduces the changes associated with the perception of an old voice.[46,53] Healthy, fit singers are able to maintain a stable fundamental frequency, intensity range, and vocal quality well into the seventh decade, indicating that physiologic age is more predictive of vocal performance than chronologic age.

The singing voice specialist works with the speech–language pathologist in caring for both singers and nonsingers.[54] The reason is that singing expands an individual's phonatory limits, increasing breath support and phrase length, increasing frequency and intensity ranges, and strengthening the voice beyond the level necessary for even extended speech. The combination of traditional voice therapy and specialized singing exercises expedites and improves outcomes in older patients.

Since 1995, the value of including an acting voice trainer in the voice team has been recognized.[55] Acting voice trainers teach techniques not only for the development of speaking voice strength and projection, but also for the control of face and body function, phonatory expression of emotion, preparation and interpretation of spoken materials, and other communication skills. Learning these techniques improves voice quality and vocal authority, thereby increasing the patient confidence in his or her ability to control vocal communication.

Surgery

In some patients with pronounced glottal incompetence, even the best voice therapy is not sufficient to overcome presbyphonia. In these cases, surgery should be considered. Vocal fold augmentation can easily be performed as an office procedure with commercially available substances such as hyaluronic acid and calcium hydroxylapatite. Thyroplasty is generally performed in the operating room under local anesthesia.

In a study by Davids and colleagues,[1] geriatric patients accounted for 21% of referrals. In this older group, the most common diagnoses were vocal fold atrophy in almost 25.0%, neurologic vocal dysfunction in 23.0%, and vocal fold immobility in 23.1%.[1] The management options offered to patients with vocal fold atrophy consisted of reassurance, voice therapy, injection laryngoplasty, and thyroplasty. Almost 40% of patients were reassured and decided to forego additional treatment. Fifty-seven percent elected to undergo voice therapy, with a statistically significant improvement in VRQOL scores after treatment. The much smaller proportion of patients who chose injection laryngoplasty also had significant improvement in VRQOL scores. These results indicate that the voice changes associated with vocal fold atrophy in geriatric patients can be treated effectively with the simple interventions of voice therapy, injection laryngoplasty, or a combination of both.

SPECIAL CONSIDERATIONS: THE UNTRAINED PROFESSIONAL SINGER AND THE CHORAL SINGER

Older, untrained professional singers present special challenges. If they have had successful careers, in many cases they have been singing correctly "naturally," despite the lack of formal training. With age, they may inadvertently adopt a poor technique in an attempt to compensate for physiologic changes. This compensation results in impaired performance ability, and increases the risk of vocal injury. Helping such singers is relatively easy, beginning with medical evaluation, followed by aerobic and physical conditioning, as well as vocal reeducation by an expert team.

The majority of people who sing are choral singers. They are devoted, enthusiastic, and commonly untrained. Unfortunately, a great many choral conductors also are untrained in voice or in vocal technique and vocal health.[56] Choral singers (regardless of age) can be helped through individual singing lessons and must be trained specifically to avoid singing too loudly because of the Lombard effect experienced in noisy choral environments. Singers should not be hoarse after rehearsals. Rather, their voices should be clear and, if anything, more "warmed up" after the rehearsal than they were at the beginning.

SUMMARY

Dysphonia in geriatric patients is common and is expected to increase as demographics continue to shift to an older population. The etiology is often multifactorial, with presbylarynx being a diagnosis of exclusion. Older voices are typically hoarse, weak, breathy, unsteady, and tremulous. Examination may reveal prominent vocal processes, atrophic vocal folds, and a spindle-shaped glottic gap. Presbyphonia is associated with depression, anxiety, social isolation, and a decreased quality of life. Histologic changes have been demonstrated in the mucosa, lamina propria, and musculature of aged vocal folds. Similar age-related changes in limb skeletal muscles of elderly patients occur as well. Convincing evidence has shown that many of these changes can be reversed or avoided with the maintenance of good general health and conditioning through regular physical exercise. Older singers are perceived to have younger voices compared with elderly nonsingers, presumably because of the benefits of regular vocal exercise. Voice exercise programs in elderly patients with age-related dysphonia provide an effective and noninvasive means of treatment, with a positive impact on quality of life, as well as improvements in acoustic measures, maximum phonation time, and vocal intensity. In selected patients, laryngeal surgery can be beneficial.

REFERENCES

1. Davids T, Klein AM, Johns MM 3rd. Current dysphonia trends in patients over the age of 65: is vocal atrophy becoming more prevalent? Laryngoscope 2012;122:332–5.
2. Roy N, Stemple J, Merrill RM, et al. Epidemiology of voice disorders in the elderly: preliminary findings. Laryngoscope 2007;117:628–33.
3. Takano S, Kimura M, Nito T, et al. Clinical analysis of presbylarynx–vocal fold atrophy in elderly individuals. Auris Nasus Larynx 2010;37:461–4.
4. Cohen SM, Turley R. Coprevalence and impact of dysphonia and hearing loss in the elderly. Laryngoscope 2009;119:1870–3.
5. Roy N, Merrill RM, Gray SD, et al. Voice disorders in the general population: prevalence, risk factors, and occupational impact. Laryngoscope 2005;115:1988–95.

6. Gregory ND, Chandran S, Lurie D, et al. Voice disorders in the elderly. J Voice 2012;26:254–8.
7. Kahane J. Anatomic and physiologic changes in the aging peripheral speech mechanism. In: Beasley DS, Davis GA, editors. Aging communication processes and disorders. New York: Grune & Stratton; 1981. p. 21–45.
8. Dhar S, Shastri S, Lenora R. Aging and the respiratory system. Med Clin North Am 1976;60:1121–39.
9. McKeown F. Pathology of the aged. London: Butterworths; 1965.
10. Mahler D. Pulmonary aspects of aging. In: Gambert SR, editor. Contemporary geriatric medicine, vol. 1. New York: Plenum Medical Book Company; 1983. p. 45–85.
11. Crapo R. The aging lung. In: Mahler DA, editor. Pulmonary disease in the elderly patient. New York: Dekker; 1993. p. 353–65.
12. Linville SE. Vocal aging. Albany (NY): Delmar Thomson Learning; 2001.
13. Sataloff RT, Linville SE. The effects of age on the voice. In: Sataloff RT, editor. Professional voice: the science and art of clinical care. 3rd edition. San Diego (CA): Plural Publishing, Inc; 2005. p. 497–511.
14. Hirano M, Kuritat S, Sakaguchi S. Ageing of the vibratory tissue of human vocal folds. Acta Otolaryngol 1989;107:428–33.
15. Ishii K, Zhai W, Akita M, et al. Ultrastructure of the lamina propria of the human vocal fold. Acta Otolaryngol 1996;116:778–82.
16. Pontes P, Brasolotto A, Behlau M. Glottic characteristics and voice complaint in the elderly. J Voice 2005;19:84–94.
17. Hirano M, Sato K, Nakashima T. Growth, development, and aging of human vocal folds. In: Bless DM, Abbs JH, editors. Vocal fold physiology. San Diego (CA): College-Hill; 1983. p. 22–43.
18. Gorham-Rowan MM, Laures-Gore J. Acoustic-perceptual correlates of voice quality in elderly men and women. J Commun Dis 2006;39:171–84.
19. Malinowski A. Shape, dimensions and process of calcification of the cartilaginous framework of the larynx in relation to age and sex in the Polish population. Folia Morphol (Warsz) 1967;26:118–28.
20. Roncollo P. Researches about ossification and conformation of the thyroid cartilage in sex and certain other factors. Mayo Clin Proc 1949;31:47–52.
21. Kahane J. Age-related changes in the peripheral speech mechanism: structural and physiological changes. Proceedings of the research symposium on communicative sciences and disorders and aging. ASHA Reports, vol. 19. Rockville (MD): American Speech Language Hearing Association; 1990. p. 75–87.
22. Thomas LB, Harrison AL, Stemple JC. Aging thyroarytenoid and limb skeletal muscle: lessons in contrast. J Voice 2008;22:430–50.
23. Lasker F. The age factor in bodily measurements of adult male and female Mexicans. Hum Biol 1953;25:50–63.
24. Levesque J, Coruff P, De Rigal J, et al. In vivo studies of the evaluation of physical properties of the human skin and aging. Int J Dermatol 1984;23:322–9.
25. Pitanguy I. Ancillary procedures in face lifting. Clin Plast Surg 1978;5:51–70.
26. Akerman S, Rohlin M, Kopp S. Bilateral degenerative changes and eviation in form of temporomandibular joints: an autopsy study of elderly individuals. Acta Odontol Scand 1984;42:205–14.
27. Nannmark U, Sennerby L, Haraldson T. Macroscopic, microscopic and radiologic assessment of the condylar part of the TMJ in elderly subjects: an autopsy study. Swed Dent J 1990;14:163–9.

28. Pereira F, Lundh H, Westesson P. Age-related changes of the retrodiscal tissues in the temporomandibular joint. J Oral Maxillofac Surg 1996;54:55–61.

29. Stratmann U, Schaarschmidt K, Santamaria P. Morphometric investigation of condylar cartilage and disc thickness in the human temporomandibular joint: significance for the definition of osteoarthritic changes. J Oral Pathol Med 1996;25:200–5.

30. DeBont L, Boering G, Liem R, et al. Osteoarthritis and internal derangement of the temporomandibular joint: a light microscopic study. J Oral Maxillofac Surg 1986;44:634–43.

31. Sonies B. The aging oropharyngeal system. In: Ripich D, editor. Handbook of geriatric communication disorders. Austin (TX): Pro-ed; 1991. p. 187–203.

32. Adams D. Age changes in oral structures. Dent Update 1991;18:14–7.

33. Klein D. Oral soft tissue changes in geriatric patients. Bull N Y Acad Med 1980;45:721–7.

34. Sasaki M. Histomorphometric analysis of age-related changes in epithelial thickness and Langerhans cell density of the human tongue. Tohoku J Exp Med 1994;173:321–36.

35. Kiuchi S, Sasaki J, Arai T, et al. Functional disorders of the pharynx and esophagus. Acta Otolaryngol Suppl 1969;256:1–30.

36. Tomoda T, Morii S, Yamashita T, et al. Histology of human eustachian tube muscles: effect of aging. Ann Otol Rhinol Laryngol 1984;93:17–24.

37. Zaino C, Benventaon T. Functional, involutional and degenerative disorders. In: Zaino C, Benventano T, editors. Radiographic examination of the oropharynx and esophagus. New York: Springer-Verlag; 1977. p. 141–76.

38. Vissink A, Spijkervet F, Amerongen A. Aging and saliva: a review of the literature. Spec Care Dentist 1996;16:95–103.

39. Crow H, Ship J. Tongue strength and endurance in different aged individuals. J Gerontol A Biol Sci Med Sci 1996;51:M247–50.

40. Mueller PB. Senescence of the voice. Bulletin: Royal College of Speech and Language Therapists 1991;476:2–5.

41. Mueller PB. The aging voice. Semin Speech Lang 1997;18:159–68.

42. Brown W, Morris R, Hicks D, et al. Phonational profiles of female professional singers and nonsingers. J Voice 1993;7:219–26.

43. Brown WS Jr, Morris RJ, Hollein H, et al. Speaking fundamental frequency characteristics as a function of age and professional singing. J Voice 1991;5:310–5.

44. Ptacek PH, Sander EK, Maloney W, et al. Phonatory and related changes with advanced age. J Speech Hear Res 1966;9:353–60.

45. Morris R, Brown W. Age-related voice measures among adult women. J Voice 1987;1:38–43.

46. Prakup B. Acoustic measures of the voices of older singers and nonsingers. J Voice 2012;26(3):341–50.

47. Golub JS, Chen PH, Otto KJ, et al. Prevalence of perceived dysphonia in a geriatric population. J Am Geriatr Soc 2006;54:1736–9.

48. Mirza N, Ruiz C, Baum ED, et al. The prevalence of major psychiatric pathologies in patients with voice disorders. Ear Nose Throat J 2003;82:808–14.

49. Sataloff RT, Sataloff J, Sokolow CJ. Hearing loss in singers and other musicians. In: Sataloff RT, editor. Professional voice: the science and art of clinical care. 3rd edition. San Diego (CA): Plural Publishing, Inc; 2005. p. 513–28.

50. Heuer RJ, Rulnick RK, Horman M, et al. Voice therapy. In: Sataloff RT, editor. Professional voice: the science and art of clinical care. 3rd edition. San Diego (CA): Plural Publishing, Inc; 2005. p. 961–86.

51. Gorman S, Weinrich B, Lee L, et al. Aerodynamic changes as a result of vocal function exercises in elderly men. Laryngoscope 2008;118:1900–3.
52. Berg EE, Hapner E, Klein A, et al. Voice therapy improves quality of life in age-related dysphonia: a case-control study. J Voice 2008;22:70–4.
53. Sataloff RT. Vocal health and pedagogy. San Diego (CA): Singular Publishing Group; 1998.
54. Sataloff RT, Baroody MM, Emerich KA, et al. The singing voice specialist. In: Sataloff RT, editor. Professional voice: the science and art of clinical care. 3rd edition. San Diego (CA): Plural Publishing, Inc; 2005. p. 1021–40.
55. Freed SL, Raphael BN, Sataloff RT. The role of the acting-voice trainer in medical care of professional voice users. In: Sataloff RT, editor. Professional voice: the science and art of clinical care. 3rd edition. San Diego (CA): Plural Publishing, Inc; 2005. p. 1051–60.
56. Sataloff RT, Smith B. Choral pedagogy. 2nd edition. San Diego (CA): Plural Publishing, Inc; 2006.

Sleep Disorders in the Elderly

Kathleen Yaremchuk, MD, MSA

KEYWORDS

- Insomnia • Sleep-disordered breathing • Sleep–wake disturbances
- Sleep fragmentation • Advanced sleep phase disorder • REM behavior disorder
- Restless leg syndrome • Periodic limb movements

KEY POINTS

- More than one-half of elderly patients report a sleep complaint—some are physiologic and others are associated with primary and secondary sleep disorders.
- Some of the issues can be improved through patient education and guidance, and others require further testing or referral for accurate diagnosis and treatment.
- It is important to recognize and give advice regarding sleep disorders to improve the quality of life and safety for the elderly and their families.

INTRODUCTION

Sleep complaints are common and reported by more than one-half of elderly patients. Many changes are physiologic, such as an increased time to fall asleep and decreased total sleep time. These changes are associated with the normal aging process. Other conditions such as sleep-disordered breathing (SDB), insomnia, sleep–wake disturbances (advance sleep phase), and movement disorders (restless leg syndrome [RLS] and periodic limb movement) should be evaluated and treated appropriately. These are primary sleep disorders that have shown an increased incidence in the elderly.

Secondary sleep disorders result from comorbid conditions that impact sleep, such as chronic pain disorders, gastroesophageal reflux, frequent urination, or dyspnea owing to congestive heart failure, chronic obstructive pulmonary disease, or asthma.

Some complaints can be improved through patient education and guidance, whereas others require testing or referral for an accurate diagnosis. It is important to recognize and give advice regarding sleep disorders to improve the quality of life and safety for the elderly and their families.

Disclosure Statement: The author has no personal financial relationships with any commercial company in the subject matter or materials discussed in this article.
Department of Otolaryngology Head and Neck Surgery, Henry Ford Hospital, 2799 West Grand Boulevard, Detroit, MI 48202, USA
E-mail address: Kyaremc1@hfhs.org

The evaluation of a patient complaining of issues of any sleep condition begins with a complete history of the patient's complaint. The use of a standardized history is helpful in gathering important information, such as duration of sleep complaints, sleep habits, and any medical conditions that may impact sleep, such as benign prostatic hypertrophy in males resulting in frequent trips to the bathroom owing to nocturia. It is also important to differentiate unrefreshing sleep from fatigue and excessive daytime somnolence. One way to think about the difference is that an individual who sits on the couch and does not want to get up to do the laundry may be fatigued, whereas the individual who falls asleep on the coach is sleepy.

NORMAL PHYSIOLOGIC CHANGES IN SLEEP PATTERNS

When evaluating sleep patterns, several parameters must be considered including the amount of sleep needed and the percentage of time spent in different sleep stages. Significant changes occur in sleep during infancy, childhood, adolescence, adulthood, and in the elderly in terms of sleep onset, sleep efficiency, and quality of sleep. These changes are considered normal and should not be a reason by themselves for concern.

The aging process brings a decrease in sleep duration. Whereas teenagers may require 9 to 10 hours of sleep a night, the elderly should expect to sleep about 7 hours. Although 8 hours of sleep a night is the norm, humans revert to an average sleep time of 7 hours 15 minutes when left in a room without environmental signals regarding light/dark, social cues, or a clock to tell time. As in all normative measurements, some individuals will sleep slightly more and others slightly less. **Fig. 1**[1] shows normal sleep stages during different periods of life.

The quality of sleep changes as well with aging. Sleep efficiency is the actual sleep time divided by time spent in bed. Sleep efficiency decreases as we age, which means that an individual will spend more time in bed but less time sleeping. Interestingly, sleep deprivation in the elderly has less impact on performance than in younger individuals.

Sleep is characterized as N1, N2, N3, and rapid eye movement (REM). N1 and N2 are considered light sleep, a period where an individual is easily awoken by noises or other interruptions. N3 and REM are considered deep sleep or "slow wave" sleep. REM sleep is when dreams occur. Part of the aging process is an increase in light sleep at the expense of deep sleep. Older individuals are more easily aroused from sleep by auditory stimuli.[2] When an arousal during sleep occurs, an individual may complain of difficulty falling back asleep. This pattern can be described as sleep fragmentation and results in lower sleep efficiency. Although it is a normal part of the aging process, it is a change and older patients can find it frustrating. Among men, sleep time decreased an average of 27 minutes per decade from midlife until the age of 80.[3] The changes in sleep patterns are more pronounced in men, but women are more likely to seek treatment and use pharmacologic agents to improve sleep quality.

Often the elderly no longer have a set schedule that requires them to go to sleep or wake up at a certain time. It is easy to overestimate or underestimate the time spent in bed or total sleep time. With complaints of difficulty falling or staying asleep, the patient should be instructed to keep a sleep diary daily for 2 weeks (**Box 1**).[4] If the individual goes to bed at 8 PM and complains of early morning awakening at 4 AM, this should not be a surprise. They are receiving their 8 hours of sleep and should consider a later bed time. The question to ask is what time does the individual want to wake up, then count back 7.5 hours to find the appropriate bed time. To fall asleep usually requires about 15 minutes in bed; greater than 30 minutes borders on abnormal.

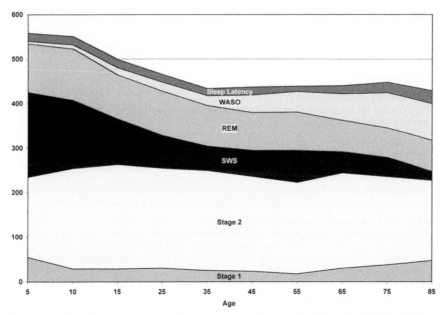

Fig. 1. Age-related trends for stage 1 sleep, stage 2 sleep, slow wave sleep (SWS), rapid eye movement (REM) sleep, wake after sleep onset (WASO), and sleep latency (in minutes). (*From* Ohayon MM, Carskadon MA, Guilleminault C, et al. Meta-analysis of quantitative sleep parameters from childhood to old age in healthy individuals: developing normative sleep values across the human lifespan. Sleep 2004;27:1270; with permission.)

Giving guidance on sleep hygiene can be helpful in this situation. **Fig. 2** lists simple steps to help improve sleep by minimizing behaviors that can be disruptive to sleep. The decrease in sleep efficiency and increase in sleep fragmentation can result in excessive daytime sleepiness (EDS) or fatigue.

The Epworth Sleepiness Scale,[5] a validated questionnaire, may be used for accurate assessment of EDS (**Fig. 3**) and to determine the likelihood of falling asleep under certain circumstances. A score of 10 or greater indicates that EDS is present and further evaluation for a cause is necessary. Some, but not all, patients with SDB often report EDS as their first symptom. The use of the Epworth Sleepiness Scale as a part of a patient's evaluation for a sleep disorder is important in recognizing the severity of the condition and the risk to the individual and others in terms of falling asleep while driving or performing other activities.

COMMON SLEEP DISORDERS IN THE ELDERLY
Advance Sleep Phase

As part of aging, a common change in the circadian rhythm is termed advance sleep phase. Advance sleep phase in the elderly may be due to changes in the suprachiasmatic nucleus, which regulates the circadian rhythm.[6] The work-retired elderly begin to go to bed earlier in the evening, such as at 8 to 9 PM, because there is little for them to do at that time of day, and subsequently experience early morning awakening at 3 to 4 AM. They find it difficult to return to sleep and complain bitterly about what they perceive to be poor sleep, when in fact they are receiving an adequate amount of sleep. Because they no longer have to get up early and be ready for their jobs, it is

Box 1
Get better sleep

Getting good sleep is important in maintaining health. There are several things that you can do to promote good sleep and sleep hygiene, and ultimately Get Better Sleep.

What is sleep hygiene?

Maintain a regular sleep routine
- Go to bed at the same time. Wake up at the same time. Ideally, your schedule will remain the same (± 20 minutes) every night of the week.

Avoid naps if possible
- Naps decrease the "sleep debt" that is so necessary for easy sleep onset.
- Each of us needs a certain amount of sleep per 24-hour period. We need that amount, and we do not need more than that.
- When we take naps, it decreases the amount of sleep that we need the next night, which may cause sleep fragmentation and difficulty initiating sleep, and may lead to insomnia.

Do not stay in bed awake for more than 30 minutes.
- If you find your mind racing, or worrying about not being able to sleep during the middle of the night, get out of bed, and sit in a chair in the dark. Do your mind racing in the chair until you are sleepy, then return to bed. No TV or Internet use during these periods! That will just stimulate you more than desired.
- If this happens several times during the night, that is OK. Just maintain your regular wake time, and try to avoid naps.

Do not watch TV or read in bed.
- When you watch TV or read in bed, you associate the bed with wakefulness.
- The bed is reserved for 2 things – sleep and hanky panky.

Drink caffeinated drinks with caution
- The effects of caffeine may last for several hours after ingestion. Caffeine can fragment sleep, and cause difficulty falling sleep. If you drink caffeine, use it only before noon.
- Remember that soda and tea contain caffeine as well.

Avoid inappropriate substances that interfere with sleep
- Cigarettes, alcohol, and over-the-counter medications may cause fragmented sleep.

Exercise regularly
- Exercise before 2 PM every day. Exercise promotes continuous sleep.
- Avoid rigorous exercise before bedtime. Rigorous exercise circulates endorphins into the body, which may cause difficulty initiating sleep.

Have a quiet, comfortable bedroom
- Set your bedroom thermostat at a comfortable temperature. Generally, a little cooler is better than a little warmer.
- Turn off the TV and other extraneous noise that may disrupt sleep. Background "white noise" like a fan is OK.
- If your pets awaken you, keep them outside the bedroom.
- Your bedroom should be dark. Turn off bright lights.

If you are a "clock watcher" at night, hide the clock.

Have a comfortable prebedtime routine
- A warm bath or shower
- Meditation or quiet time

From American Sleep Association. Get better sleep. Available at: https://www.sleepassociation.org/get-better-sleep/. Accessed October 20, 2017; with permission.

difficult for them to break the habit of going to bed early without some guidance. Bright light therapy or being outside in the daylight in the late afternoon can help to "reset" their clock to a more socially acceptable sleep schedule.[7] Changing a sleep schedule is not easy and cannot occur overnight. When sleep–wake times are changed, for

Consensus Sleep Diary-M (Please Complete Upon Awakening)   ID/NAME: _____
Sample

Today's Date	4/5/11							
1. What time did you get into bed?	10:15 p.m.							
2. What time did you try to go to sleep?	11:30 p.m.							
3. How long did it take you to fall asleep?	55 min.							
4. How many times did you wake up, not counting your final awakening?	6 times							
5. In total, how long did these awakenings last?	2 h 5 min.							
6a. What time was your final awakening?	6:35 a.m.							
6b. After your final awakening, how long did you spend in bed trying to sleep?	45 min.							
6c. Did you wake up earlier than you planned?	☒ Yes ☐ No	☐ Yes ☐ No	☐ Yes ☐ No	☐ Yes ☐ No	☐ Yes ☐ No	☐ Yes ☐ No	☐ Yes ☐ No	☐ Yes ☐ No
6d. If yes, how much earlier?	1 h							
7. What time did you get out of bed for the day?	7:20 a.m.							
8. In total, how long did you sleep?	4 h 10 min.							
9. How would you rate the quality of your sleep?	☐ Very poor ☒ Poor ☐ Fair ☐ Good ☐ Very good	☐ Very poor ☐ Poor ☐ Fair ☐ Good ☐ Very good	☐ Very poor ☐ Poor ☐ Fair ☐ Good ☐ Very good	☐ Very poor ☐ Poor ☐ Fair ☐ Good ☐ Very good	☐ Very poor ☐ Poor ☐ Fair ☐ Good ☐ Very good	☐ Very poor ☐ Poor ☐ Fair ☐ Good ☐ Very good	☐ Very poor ☐ Poor ☐ Fair ☐ Good ☐ Very good	☐ Very poor ☐ Poor ☐ Fair ☐ Good ☐ Very good
10. How rested or refreshed did you feel when you woke-up for the day?	☐ Not at all rested ☒ Slightly rested ☐ Somewhat rested ☐ Well-rested ☐ Very well-rested	☐ Not at all rested ☐ Slightly rested ☐ Somewhat rested ☐ Well-rested ☐ Very well-rested	☐ Not at all rested ☐ Slightly rested ☐ Somewhat rested ☐ Well-rested ☐ Very well-rested	☐ Not at all rested ☐ Slightly rested ☐ Somewhat rested ☐ Well-rested ☐ Very well-rested	☐ Not at all rested ☐ Slightly rested ☐ Somewhat rested ☐ Well-rested ☐ Very well-rested	☐ Not at all rested ☐ Slightly rested ☐ Somewhat rested ☐ Well-rested ☐ Very well-rested	☐ Not at all rested ☐ Slightly rested ☐ Somewhat rested ☐ Well-rested ☐ Very well-rested	☐ Not at all rested ☐ Slightly rested ☐ Somewhat rested ☐ Well-rested ☐ Very well-rested

Fig. 2. Sleep diary instructions (CSD-M). (*From* Carney CE, Buysse DJ, Ancoli-Israel S, et al. The consensus sleep diary: standardizing prospective sleep self-monitoring. Sleep 2012;35:295.)

example, as a result of daylight savings time, the loss of an hour of sleep results in an increase in motor vehicle accidents. It usually takes 1 week for an individual to adjust to a 1-hour change in a bedtime sleep time.

Owing to early morning awakenings, it is not uncommon for the elderly to become sleepy and nap midday, which is when we all have a circadian rhythm-induced dip in alertness. Studies have shown that naps in the elderly resulted in an increase in 24-hour sleep amounts and enhanced cognitive and psychomotor performance immediately after the nap and throughout the next day.[8]

Sleep-Disordered Breathing

SDB is a spectrum of disorders defined by the pressure that causes inspiratory airflow to cease. Normal breathing, snoring, obstructive hypopneas, and obstructive apneas during sleep each may begin with a complaint of snoring by a spouse and ultimately be diagnosed from a sleep study as obstructive sleep apnea (OSA). OSA is a highly prevalent disease with an increasing incidence because of an epidemic of obesity in the population. In older adults, rates range from 38% to more than 60%.[9]

Characterized by recurrent episodes of upper airway obstructions that cause decreased ventilation and oxygen desaturations, OSA is associated with an increase in cardiovascular and cerebrovascular morbidity and mortality. Evidence has shown that the presence of SDB in the elderly is associated with cognitive impairment. The major risk factors for the disorder are obesity, male gender, postmenopausal status, and age. A body mass index of 30 kg/m^2 or greater with a neck circumference of 17 inches or greater in a male and 14.5 inches or greater in a female indicates a 70% chance of being diagnosed with OSA.

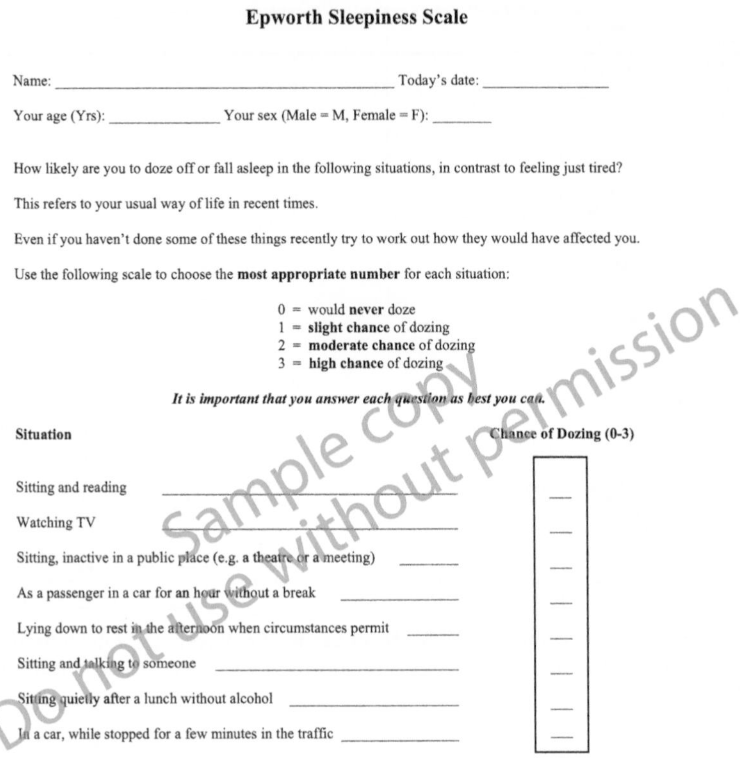

Epworth Sleepiness Scale

Name: _____ Today's date: _____

Your age (Yrs): _____ Your sex (Male = M, Female = F): _____

How likely are you to doze off or fall asleep in the following situations, in contrast to feeling just tired?

This refers to your usual way of life in recent times.

Even if you haven't done some of these things recently try to work out how they would have affected you.

Use the following scale to choose the **most appropriate number** for each situation:

0 = would **never** doze
1 = **slight chance** of dozing
2 = **moderate chance** of dozing
3 = **high chance** of dozing

It is important that you answer each question as best you can.

Situation   **Chance of Dozing (0-3)**

Sitting and reading _____   ___

Watching TV _____   ___

Sitting, inactive in a public place (e.g. a theatre or a meeting) _____   ___

As a passenger in a car for an hour without a break _____   ___

Lying down to rest in the afternoon when circumstances permit _____   ___

Sitting and talking to someone _____   ___

Sitting quietly after a lunch without alcohol _____   ___

In a car, while stopped for a few minutes in the traffic _____   ___

Fig. 3. Epworth sleepiness scale. (ESS © MW Johns 1990-1997. Used under License. Contact information and permission to use: Mapi Research Trust, Lyon, France. – Internet: https://eprovide.mapi-trust.org.)

The classic signs and symptoms for OSA are upper airway obstruction during sleep, insomnia, and daytime hypersomnolence. As an individual falls asleep and muscle relaxation occurs, the upper airway obstructs and an arousal occurs with the return of a lighter sleep stage or an awakening and a subsequent increase in muscle tone to open the airway. This pattern occurs multiple times throughout the night and results in increased sleep fragmentation and unrefreshing sleep, even though sleep duration is adequate. Hypersomnolence is evident and problematic and presents quality of life as well as safety issues.

An attended sleep study or home sleep study is necessary to make the diagnosis of OSA. An attended sleep study is done in a certified sleep laboratory. Electroencephalography, electrocardiography, pulse oximetry, chest and abdominal sensors, nasal airflow and temperature, limb movements, extraocular movements, and video-recording are performed. This type of study is recommended for individuals with pulmonary, cardiovascular, and/or neurologic deficits or sleep-related movement disorders or a suspicion for narcolepsy.

Portable or home sleep studies have become more common and are usually mandated as the first line of testing by insurance companies. They are significantly less expensive and easier to obtain. For patients with suspected OSA but no significant comorbidities, a home sleep study is adequate to make a diagnosis of OSA. A portable or home sleep study will record the heart rate, oximetry, and obstructive respiratory events. The patient is given a device to use at night and return to the sleep center the next day for result reporting.

OSA is categorized as mild, moderate, or severe based on the results of the sleep study. An obstructive apnea is scored as a cessation of air flow with respiratory effort for 10 seconds, and a hypopnea is a 50% reduction of airflow with respiratory effort or a decrease in oxygen saturation of 3% and decreased respiratory effort. Medicare requires a desaturation of 4% for the scoring of a hypopnea. The apnea–hypopnea index (AHI) is the number of apneas and hypopneas per hour of sleep. An AHI of 5 to 15 is considered mild OSA, 15 to 30 is moderate OSA, and 30 or greater is considered severe OSA. The AHI requirements for diagnosis of mild, moderate, or severe OSA have changed over the years, and the research regarding the health impact of OSA can be confusing.

For patients with mild OSA, there is little evidence to support treatment without documentation of EDS based on results of Epworth Sleepiness Scale for those with diabetes or cardiovascular disease. For that reason, insurance companies often will not approve treatment of mild OSA without clinical documentation of the aforementioned conditions.

Untreated moderate and severe OSA are associated with an increased risk of death from all-cause mortality, so it is an important health risk. Research has substantiated the association of SDB and earlier cognitive decline in elderly women.[10] The presence of SDB also has shown a bidirectional relationship with Alzheimer's disease.[11]

Multiple treatment options are available for OSA. The most common first-line therapy is continuous positive airway pressure (CPAP). CPAP is a pneumatic splint that keeps the airway open by using positive airway pressure during sleep. CPAP uses a continuous pressure that may be determined through a CPAP titration study. A sleep study is performed in which the patient wears a mask with increasing pressure levels until apneas are eliminated. Because the technology has markedly improved, autopap is now prescribed once a sleep study documents the presence of OSA. Autopap responds to resistance in the airway and changes pressure based on the resistance in the airway. The devices document AHI, leaks, and usage on a daily basis and are able to transmit the data to physicians and durable medical equipment companies to document compliance, which is required by insurance companies. Masks may be full face for mouth breathers, nasal masks, or nasal pillows, which some individuals find more comfortable. Insurance requires patients to use CPAP 4 hours 70% of nights or 5 of 7 nights to meet guidelines for compliance. If patients are unable to meet the standard, insurance companies will not reimburse for the device. A problem with CPAP is compliance, with 30% to 50% of patients not tolerating the device.

Oral appliances can also be used and many individuals find them less intrusive and more comfortable than a CPAP device. Acceptance of oral appliances ranges from 67% to 100% with an average of 91%.[12] Patients that are edentulous or have temporomandibular joint problems may not be able to use oral appliances.

Surgical options are also available for treatment of patients with OSA. Uvulopalatopharyngoplasty with or without tonsillectomy, genioglossal advancement, and maxillomandibular advancement are a few of the surgical procedures used for OSA. Elderly surgical candidates do well; there is no evidence that surgery should not be considered in this group.

The hypoglossal nerve implant was approved by the US Food and Drug Administration in 2014 and has no upper age restriction. It is indicated for patients who have tried and failed CPAP and/or traditional upper airway surgeries. The implantable device stimulates the hypoglossal nerve to extend the tongue and open the airway in conjunction with respiratory effort.

In obese patients with OSA, weight loss can have significant impact. A 10% loss of total body weight can result in a 27% decrease in AHI. Exercise has also shown to be helpful by increasing muscle tone. Daily exercise without a change in body mass index can result in a decrease in the AHI.

Insomnia

Insomnia is the most common form of sleep disturbance. Insomnia is described as a persistent difficulty initiating or maintaining sleep that results in general sleep dissatisfaction. The sleep complaint is accompanied by distress about poor sleep and/or impairment in family, social, vocational, academic, or other important areas of functioning. For an insomnia diagnosis, the individual must have difficulty with sleep latencies and periods of wakefulness during sleep greater than 30 minutes at least 3 times a week. If the complaints are present for less than 3 months, it is termed short-term insomnia disorder; if the symptoms have been present for more than 3 months, it is considered a chronic insomnia disorder. Chronic insomnia disorder occurs in about 10% of the population and women are more likely to be seen for this complaint. It may occur at any age, but is more commonly diagnosed in older adults, most likely owing to an age-related deterioration in sleep continuity and an increase in medical comorbidities and use of medications that increase insomnia risk.[13] Elderly patients are frequently on medications that can disrupt sleep and cause insomnia (**Table 1**).

SDB and advance phase shift can often be the cause of insomnia. As discussed elsewhere in this article, these conditions should be ruled out through a sleep study or a careful sleep history. A polysomnogram or sleep study is not indicated for diagnosis of insomnia.

A sleep diary will help by letting the clinician know if the patient is going to bed too early and thus frustrated by early morning awakenings or just not achieving 7 hours of sleep a night. Naps can interfere with normal sleep if the number of naps or time spent napping is excessive. A refreshing power nap of 20 to 60 minutes in the afternoon will not be problematic, but several naps of 2 to 3 hours will deplete the need for 7 hours of sleep at night. Completion of a sleep diary can be helpful in making the correct diagnosis (see **Box 1**).[4]

Some elderly patients become sedentary and spend much of their time in bed watching television or reading. Some will even have their meals in bed. The bed becomes an office, kitchen, and entertainment area that is no longer strictly associated with sleep. For that reason, it is recommended that individuals only use the bed for sleep and sex and not keep the television on to help them fall asleep.

Clock watching is another pattern that causes anxiety during the night. The normal sleep cycle is 90 minutes long, and starts with wakefulness, transitions from light to deep sleep, and then dreaming with REM sleep. After 90 minutes of sleep, it is not unusual for an individual to have an "arousal" when entering the lighter sleep phase. If they look at the clock, they may start to calculate how much time they have before they need to get out of bed, which in turn may cause a fully awake state and require another 30 minutes to fall asleep. This pattern causes decreased sleep efficiency and increased sleep fragmentation. This type of insomnia is characterized as sleep maintenance insomnia or the inability to fall back asleep after normal sleep onset. Explaining the normal sleep pattern of a 90-minute cycle and asking patients to turn the clock away from themselves to stop the habit can be helpful. Depression can also be a factor with insomnia and should be considered as a cause as well and treated to improve the insomnia.

If insomnia is persistent, cognitive behavioral therapy (CBT) or medication should be considered. CBT for insomnia (CBT-I) is a technique for treating insomnia without (or alongside) medications. CBT-I aims to improve sleep habits and behaviors by

Table 1
Medications and their effects on sleep

Medication	Examples	Sleep
Antiarrhythmics	Procainamide (Procanbid), quinidine (Cardioquin), disopyramide (Norpace)	Nighttime sleep difficulties, daytime fatigue
Beta-blockers	Atenolol (Tenormin), metoprolol (Lopressor), propranolol (Inderal)	Insomnia, nighttime awakenings, nightmares
Clonidine	High blood pressure; sometimes prescribed off-label for alcohol withdrawal or smoking cessation	Daytime drowsiness and fatigue, disrupted REM sleep; less commonly, restlessness, early morning awakening, nightmares
Corticosteroids	Prednisone (Sterapred, others)	Daytime jitters, insomnia
Diuretics	Chlorothiazide (Diuril), chlorthalidone (Hygroton), hydrochlorothiazide (Esidrix, HydroDIURIL, others)	Increased nighttime urination, painful calf cramps during sleep
Medications containing alcohol	Coricidin HBP, Nyquil Cough, Theraflu Warming Relief	Suppressed REM sleep, disrupted nighttime sleep
Nicotine replacement products	Nicotine patches (Nicoderm), gum (Nicorette), nasal spray or inhalers (Nicotrol), and lozenges (Commit)	Insomnia, disturbing dreams
Selective serotonin reuptake inhibitors	Fluoxetine (Prozac), sertraline (Zoloft), paroxetine (Paxil)	Decreased REM sleep, daytime fatigue
Bronchodilators	Theophylline (Slo-bid, Theo-Dur, others)	Wakefulness similar to that caused by caffeine
Thyroid hormone	Levothyroxine (Levoxyl, Synthroid, others)	Sleeping difficulties (at higher doses)

Abbreviation: REM, rapid eye movement.

identifying and changing the thoughts and behaviors that affect the ability to allow the person to sleep or sleep well. CBT-I usually consists of 4 to 6 sessions of 30 to 60 minutes in duration. CBT is designed to correct misconceptions about the effects of aging on sleep, improve sleep hygiene, and develop strategies to overcome the worry and other negative emotions that accompany the experience of being unable to sleep. Studies have shown marked improvement in individuals who have completed CBT-I that is sustainable compared with individuals who use sleep-promoting medications. Those who use sleep-promoting medications were found to return to baseline, whereas individuals who received CBT-I showed continued improvement for 6 months after therapy.[14]

The use of sleep-promoting medications has been associated with dependence and falls in the elderly when getting up at night to go to the bathroom. A strong association has been found with certain pharmacologic sleep aids and compulsive gambling, eating, or shopping behaviors. The need for adequate sleep in the elderly needs to be balanced with possible health risks and safety.

Sleep-Related Movement Disorders

RLS is an uncontrollable urge to move the legs when sitting or lying down. The symptoms are characterized by the acronym "URGE":

- *U*rge to move the legs, usually associated with unpleasant leg sensations;
- *R*est induces symptoms;
- *G*etting active brings relief; and
- *E*vening and night makes symptoms worse.

RLS is a clinical diagnosis, occurs in 10% of the population, and generally worsens as one ages. The individual describes the sensation as a deep-seated discomfort that is usually below the knees. The sensation is described as a crawling, creeping, pulling, aching, itching, drawing, or stretching. Movement of the legs immediately relieves the sensation, but it returns when the legs become still again.

RLS is associated with iron deficiency, end-stage renal disease, diabetes, multiple sclerosis, Parkinson's disease, and pregnancy. A family history of RLS is common; pedigrees in these cases suggest an autosomal-dominant transmission with high penetrance.[15]

According to a commonly held view, RLS may be due to dysfunction of dopamine cells in the nigrostriatal areas of the brain. Pharmacologic studies have shown a dramatic improvement of RLS symptoms with the administration of levodopa, the precursor of dopamine, or with dopaminergic agonists acting on dopamine receptors in the brain.

It is recommended that ferritin levels be checked in patients with RLS. Recent research suggests that an iron deficiency in the area of the brain responsible for dopaminergic production that may not improve with oral iron supplementation. Iron is a necessary cofactor in the brain for the synthesis of dopamine and the regulation of dopamine receptors, and for dopamine available in the synapse. Iron and ferritin have been found to be abnormally low in the cerebrospinal fluid of patients with RLS. Iron supplementation is recommended in the presence of low serum ferritin, but even with normal serum ferritin an iron deficiency may exist in the brain that is responsible for RLS.

The need to ambulate to relieve the symptoms of RLS results in sleep fragmentation and decreased sleep time. RLS is a major cause of insomnia because individuals cannot fall asleep owing to leg discomfort or because they wake up with the need to ambulate to relieve the symptoms.

First-line treatment for RLS involves dopaminergic agents, including dopamine agonists and levodopa. Dopamine agonists such as pramipexole, ropinirole, and rotigotine are generally more effective than levodopa, but are associated with more side effects. In patients with iron deficiency, iron supplementation is an important component of treatment.

Periodic Limb Movement

Periodic limb movement disorder (PLMD) is characterized by repeated leg jerks or kicks during sleep that are accompanied by clinical sleep disturbance or fatigue. Similar movements can occur in the upper extremities. The bed partner will complain of being hit or kicked, and the individual will have no awareness of the movement. Whereas patients with RLS experience their symptoms during wakefulness, PLMD occurs during sleep. About 80% of patients with RLS will have PLMD. There is significant overlap between the 2 conditions, but only about 20% of those with PLMD report RLS. About 45% of elderly patients have PLMD compared with 5% to 6% in younger individuals.

Dopaminergic deficiency has been implicated in PLMD and treatment is with dopaminergic agents, much like with RLS.[16] If the individual does not complain of a clinical sleep disturbance or fatigue, and if it is only the bed partner is bothered by the movements, pharmacologic treatment is not recommended owing to possible side effects.

Rapid Eye Movement Sleep Behavior Disorder

REM sleep behavior disorder (RBD) is technically a parasomnia but is characterized by movement during REM sleep.[17] REM sleep results in muscle atonia and is often termed an awake brain in an asleep body. In RBD, however, the individual has muscle tone and is able to act out their dreams. Bed partners describe the individual engaging in purposeful violent movement such as kicking, punching, or leaping from the bed. Sleep-related injury to the individual or the bed partner is common. At the end of an episode or when awoken by the bed partner, the individual can report a dream that describes being chased or attacked by a force that they need to defend themselves against.

RDB is a male-predominant disorder that usually occurs after 50 years of age. There may be an underlying neurologic disorder, such as Parkinson disease, multiple system atrophy, dementia with Lewy bodies, narcolepsy, or stroke. A sleep study is necessary to make the diagnosis of RBD. The sleep study demonstrates muscle tone during REM sleep, which is abnormal. Eliminating other sleep disorders such as SDB is important because they can exacerbate RBD.

This disorder is particularly frightening for bed partners because they are often the target of the violent movements. Safety for the individual and bed partner is important. Clonazepam is suggested for the treatment of RBD, but should be used with caution in patients with dementia, gait disorders, or concomitant OSA owing to its sedative effects. More recently, melatonin has been recommended because it eliminates the concerns regarding the sedative and addictive properties of clonazepam.

SUMMARY

There are normal changes in sleep patterns in the elderly that can cause concern for individuals. Sometimes counseling and sharing of information is sufficient to alleviate concern. Multiple sleep disorders such as insomnia, SDB, and movement disorders increase in frequency as individuals age. Some of these disorders are magnified by neurologic or metabolic disorders. The otolaryngologist plays an important role in diagnosis and treatment or referral to a sleep specialist. This article was meant to help guide decision making by giving information on the most common sleep disturbances in the elderly.

REFERENCES

1. Ohayan M, Carskadon MA, Guilleminault C, et al. Meta-analysis of quantitative sleep parameters from childhood to old age in healthy individuals: developing normative sleep values across the human lifespan. Sleep 2004;27:1255–73.
2. Zepelin H, McDonald CS, Zammit GK. Effects of age on auditory awakening threshold. J Gerontol 1984;39:294–300.
3. Van Cauter EV, Leproult R, Plat L. Age-Related changes in slow wave sleep and REM sleep and relationship with growth hormone and cortisol levels in healthy men. JAMA 2000;284:861–8.
4. Carney CE, Buysse DJ, Ancoli-Israel S, et al. The consensus sleep diary: standardizing prospective sleep self-monitoring. Sleep 2012;35(2):287–302.
5. Johns MW. A new method for measuring daytime sleepiness: the Epworth sleepiness scale. Sleep 1991;14:540–5.

6. Swaab DF, Fliers E, Partiman TS. The suprochiasmatic nucleus of the human brain in relation so sex, age and senile dementia. Brain Res 1985;342:37–44.

7. Campbell SS, Terman M, Lew AJ, et al. Light treatment for sleep disorders: consensus report. Age related disturbances. J Biol Rhythms 1995;10:151–4.

8. Campbell SS, Murphy PJ, Stauble TN. Effects of a nap on nighttime sleep and waking function in older subjects. J Am Geriatr Soc 2005;53:48–53.

9. Ancoli-Israel S, Kripke D, Mason W, et al. Sleep apnea and nocturnal myoclonus in a senior population. Sleep 1981;4:486–95.

10. Spira A, Blackwell T, Stone K, et al. Sleep-disordered breathing and cognition in older women. J Am Geriatr Soc 2008;56:45–50.

11. Jo Y, Lucey B, Holtzman D. Sleep and Alzheimer disease pathology-a bidirectional relationship. Nat Rev Neurol 2014;10(2):115–9.

12. Vanderveken OM, Dieltjens M, Wouters K, et al. Objective measurement of compliance during oral appliance therapy for sleep-disordered breathing. Thorax 2013;68:91–6.

13. American Academy of Sleep Medicine. International classification of sleep disorders. 3rd edition. Darien (IL): American academy of Sleep Medicine; 2014.

14. Edinger J, Wohgemuth W, Radtke R, et al. Cognitive behavioral therapy for chronic primary insomnia a randomized controlled trial. JAMA 2001;285: 1856–64.

15. Ekbom K, Ulfberg J. Restless legs syndrome. J Intern Med 2009;266:419–31.

16. Roepke SK, Ancoli-Israel S. Sleep disorders in the elderly. Indian J Med Res 2010;131:302–10.

17. Aurora RN, Zak RS, Maganti RK, et al. Best practice guide for the treatment of REM behavior disorder (RBD). J Clin Sleep Med 2010;6(1):85–95.

Rhinosinusitis and Allergies in Elderly Patients

Constanza J. Valdés, MD[a,b], Marc A. Tewfik, MD, MSc, FRCSC[c,*]

KEYWORDS

- Rhinitis • Rhinosinusitis • Elderly • Management • Presbynasalis

KEY POINTS

- The anatomy and physiology of the sinonasal tract changes with advancing age, occasionally resulting in symptoms.
- Multiple factors in geriatric patients can lead to a decrease in olfactory function.
- The causes of rhinitis in elderly patients are variable, and treatment should be tailored to the patient's individual needs, medications, and comorbidities.
- Chronic rhinosinusitis management can be more challenging in geriatric patients because of previous treatments and surgeries.

INTRODUCTION

The elderly population has increased in developed countries and, with this, diseases in the geriatric population are becoming increasingly important. It is projected that by the year 2050, individuals older than 65 years will represent 20% of the population in the United States and 25% of the Canadian population.[1,2] Up to one-third of patients seen by an otolaryngologist are older than the age of 65 years.[3] The Canadian population has a mean life expectancy of 81 years of age[4] and they expect a good quality of life as they age.

Although evidence suggests that allergic rhinitis decreases with age, the prevalence of nonallergic rhinitis is higher in the elderly, and rhinosinusitis is the sixth most common chronic disease in the elderly population.[5] Furthermore, elderly patients are often affected by multiple comorbidities, which can be more severe than rhinitis and rhinosinusitis. Nevertheless, poorly controlled rhinitis and rhinosinusitis can act as triggers for respiratory disease exacerbation and affect the patient's quality of life, underlining the importance of assessing and treating these conditions.[6] Of course, a careful

[a] Department of Otolaryngology–Head and Neck Surgery, Hospital del Salvador, Universidad de Chile, Av. Salvador 364, Providencia, Santiago 7500922, Chile; [b] Department of Otolaryngology–Head and Neck Surgery, Clínica Las Condes, Av. Estoril 450, Las Condes, Santiago 7591047, Chile; [c] Department of Otolaryngology–Head and Neck Surgery, McGill University Health Center, 1001 Decarie Boulevard, Room D05.5718, Montreal, Québec H4A 3J1, Canada
* Corresponding author.
E-mail address: marc.tewfik@mcgill.ca

Clin Geriatr Med 34 (2018) 217–231
https://doi.org/10.1016/j.cger.2018.01.009
0749-0690/18/© 2018 Elsevier Inc. All rights reserved.

evaluation of comorbidities and potential drug interactions should be undertaken before prescribing any pharmacologic therapy.

Anatomic and Physiologic Changes with Age

Several changes in nasal physiology, anatomy, and in the immune system occur with advancing age; these changes can influence the onset of rhinitis and rhinosinusitis symptoms in older adults.

The term presbynasalis refers to the changes in the sinonasal tract that occur with age.[7] These changes involve the anatomy, the mucosa, and the viscoelastic properties of nasal secretions.

Anatomy

Fibroconnective tissues become weaker because of collagen fiber atrophy and a decrease in facial musculature; this leads to a loss of tip support and ptosis.[8] There can also be septal cartilage fragmentation and retraction of the columella. These structural changes can decrease nasal airflow and lead to symptoms of nasal obstruction.

Nasal mucosa

There is often atrophy of the nasal mucosa with advancing age caused by a thinning of both the epithelium and the basal membrane,[9] variably affecting nasal airflow and altering mucociliary clearance. These same changes are observed in postmenopausal women.[10] There is a decrease in ciliary beat frequency and mucociliary clearance[11] accompanied by alterations of the microtubules.[7,12] Nasal vasculature also changes as submucosal vessels become less patent, resulting in a decreased ability of nasal structures to warm and humidify inhaled air. Consequently, older individuals are more susceptible to suffering from nasal dryness.[13]

Viscoelastic properties of the secretions

With a decrease in the production and secretion of nasal mucous, there is an increase in the viscosity of secretions, which further contributes to the sensation of dryness and irritation.

The immune system is also affected with age, with 2 major changes noted: immunosenescence and the development of chronic inflammation.[14]

Immunosenescence describes changes in both innate and acquired immunity with age, which can cause an increased susceptibility to infections and autoimmune disorders. These changes include

1. Decreased expression and signaling of toll-like receptors[15]
2. Involution of the thymus gland, resulting in the decreased production and differentiation of naïve T cells, and a decreased responsiveness of T-cell populations[12]
3. Increased production of aberrant antibodies to pneumococcus and other bacteria by B cells.[16]

This process of immunosenescence affects the sinonasal tract, resulting in a greater vulnerability to allergens and pathogens in the elderly population.[7]

With age, the olfactory neuroepithelium also undergoes modifications: it becomes thinner, the density of receptors decreases, and the pattern of receptors changes.[17] These changes are more pronounced in smokers.[18] This results in a decreased sense of smell with age: after the age of 65 years, about 20% of patients present with alterations in their sense of smell and in patients older than 80 years up to 62.5% have alterations in olfaction.[19] There is not only a decrease in the perception of odors but also in distinguishing between different odorants.[20] This decrease adversely affects quality of life because the ability to distinguish flavors and taste diminishes.

Decreased olfaction may also present as an early symptom of neurodegenerative diseases. Loss of smell is an early symptom in Parkinson disease that is present in approximately 90% of affected patients and precedes motor symptoms by approximately 4 to 6 years. The mechanisms responsible for olfactory dysfunction are currently unknown.[21–23] It also occurs in other disorders such as Alzheimer disease, Huntington disease, and multiple sclerosis.

Although the loss of smell is frequent, only about 9% of the patients perceive and report it, putting these patients at risk for cooking mishaps, natural gas leaks, and inadvertently consuming spoiled food. In patients with allergic rhinitis, there is a decrease in olfaction that is attributed not only to obstruction but also to inflammation of the olfactory cleft.[24,25] In older adults, multiple factors often contribute to the loss of smell.

Rhinitis in the Elderly

Rhinitis is an inflammation of the nasal mucosa, characterized clinically by 1 or more of the following symptoms: nasal congestion, rhinorrhea or posterior discharge, itching of the nose and/or eyes, and sneezing. Rhinitis is a prevalent condition in the elderly and is of concern because of its relationship with asthma; it has a substantial socioeconomic cost and heavily affects quality of life. It can be classified as allergic or nonallergic (**Table 1**).

Allergic rhinitis seems to decrease with age, with a prevalence of 12%,[26] although recent literature suggests a prevalence of approximately 32%[27] in the 54 to 89 years age group. Several studies have suggested that rhinitis symptoms become milder with time and that allergic skin reactivity also decreases.[28–30] The 2005 National Center for Health Statistics Report noted the prevalence of allergic rhinitis as 7.8% in those 65 to 75 years old, and 5.4% in those older than 75 years.[31] Although there is little research regarding nonallergic rhinitis, the prevalence seems to be greater in women and seems to increase with age.[32,33]

Table 1 **Classification of rhinitis**	
Allergic	**Nonallergic**
Intermittent	Noninfectious
Persistent	Occupational
	Caused by work: symptoms arises of causes attributable to a particular work environment
	Exacerbated by work: preexisting rhinitis exacerbated in the workplace
	Drug-induced
	Various drugs (see **Table 2**)
	Medicamentosa
	Hormonal
	Hypothyroidism, acromegaly
	Idiopathic
	Vasomotor rhinitis
	Other
	Nonallergic rhinitis with eosinophilia syndrome (NARES)
	Gustatory rhinitis
	Atrophic
	Infectious
	Viral
	Adenovirus, influenza, parainfluenza
	Bacterial
	Streptococcus, hemophilus

ALLERGIC RHINITIS

Allergic rhinitis is characterized by intermittent or persistent symptoms such as rhinorrhea, nasal congestion, sneezing, itching, or pruritus.[34] These symptoms are the result of a type I hypersensitivity reaction with an immunoglobulin (Ig)E-mediated allergic inflammation in the nasal mucosa triggered by various allergens; the symptoms can be perennial or seasonal. After the cell is exposed to an allergen, it produces specific IgE antibodies directed against these extrinsic proteins that bind to the surface of mast cells. When the patient is exposed again to the allergen, the mast cells release previously formed mediators, consisting mainly of histamine, which then exert their effects on the nasal mucosa. The early phase response is immediate up to 2 hours after exposure to the antigen. It relies on preformed mediators within the sensitized mastocyte that degranulates, releasing histamine to produce symptoms. The late-phase response is produced by neoformed mediators from the mastocyte membrane, such as lipoxygenase (prostaglandins and thromboxanes), cyclooxygenase (leukotrienes), and cellular recruitment (basophils, eosinophils). These mediators will cause vascular endothelial dilation, which subsequently causes mucosal edema. This leads to the symptoms of congestion, redness, tearing, swelling, and postnasal drip. The allergen will stimulate irritant receptors, causing itching and sneezing. Both phases present similar symptoms; however, sneezing and itching are less prominent in the late phase, whereas congestion and mucus production are more severe.[35] In elderly patients, however, the late phase may be not noticed by patients due to a very limited or nonexistent course.[36]

To make a diagnosis of allergic rhinitis, there must be objective evidence of allergen sensitivity (skin test or serum testing). Allergen sensitization, as well as total IgE, seems to diminish with age. Simola and colleagues[30] showed that prick test reactivity trended down in older subjects and that there were no associations between this decrease and the duration of rhinitis symptoms or changes in symptom severity. Additionally, symptoms tended to become milder with time, independent of prick test sensitivity. A more recent study analyzed the symptoms, skin prick testing (SPT), serum total, and specific IgE and nasal eosinophils 15 years after primary testing. In 180 subjects, symptoms became milder with a decrease of specific serum IgE and nasal eosinophils, with no differences in serum IgE or SPT. They showed that the decrease in nasal symptoms was related with nasal eosinophil independently of SPT and IgE.[37] Allergic rhinitis is classified as intermittent or persistent disease and its severity as mild or moderate to severe **(Fig. 1)**.[38]

NONALLERGIC RHINITIS

Nonallergic rhinitis is also characterized by signs and symptoms of nasal inflammation but without any identifiable type 1 hypersensitivity. It can be subdivided into several categories as follows.

Idiopathic Rhinitis, Also Known as Vasomotor Rhinitis

The cause of idiopathic rhinitis is unclear but there seems to be a role for nasal inflammation, C-fibers, parasympathetic hyperreactivity, and/or sympathetic hyporeactivity, as well as glandular hyperreactivity. Patients are hyperresponsive to nonspecific environmental triggers such as changes in temperature and humidity, exposure to tobacco smoke, and strong odors. It commonly causes watery rhinorrhea, which can be unilateral or bilateral.

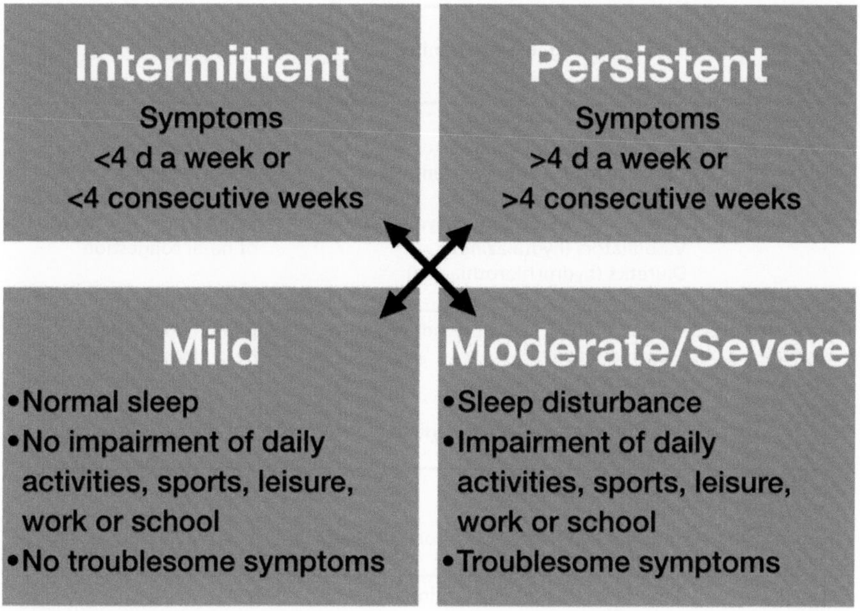

Intermittent Symptoms <4 d a week or <4 consecutive weeks	Persistent Symptoms >4 d a week or >4 consecutive weeks
Mild •Normal sleep •No impairment of daily activities, sports, leisure, work or school •No troublesome symptoms	Moderate/Severe •Sleep disturbance •Impairment of daily activities, sports, leisure, work or school •Troublesome symptoms

Fig. 1. Classification of allergic rhinitis. (*Adapted from* Bousquet J, Van Cauwenberge P, Khaltaev N. Allergic rhinitis and its impact on asthma. J Allergy Clin Immunol 2001;108(Suppl 5):S148; with permission.)

Atrophic Rhinitis

Atrophic rhinitis is a chronic disease of the nasal cavity mucosa of unknown cause. This condition is progressive and is characterized by atrophy of the nasal mucosa and the underlying bone of the turbinates, with abnormal dilatation of the nasal cavities, paradoxic nasal congestion, and formation of viscous secretions and dry crusts, leading to a characteristic fetidity, commonly called ozena.[39] Secondary atrophic rhinitis occurs as a consequence of a particular condition that acts as the main triggering factor, such as extensive nasal surgery, trauma, inflammatory processes, granulomatous diseases, or radiation therapy.

Drug-Induced Rhinitis

The symptoms of drug-induced rhinitis usually reduce sympathetic vascular tone, causing vasodilation and increased nasal congestion (**Table 2**). More than 400 brand name drugs list rhinitis as a side effect. It is of importance because of the polypharmacy often seen in the geriatric population; on average, patients older than 65 years use at least 5 medications and 12% use at least 10 medications.[40] Rhinitis medicamentosa is a persistent nasal obstruction after using nasal sympathomimetic agents due to rebound vasodilation with overuse.

Gustatory Rhinitis

Gustatory rhinitis is watery rhinorrhea after ingestion of certain foods.

EVALUATION

The evaluation of the elderly patient should include a full history of symptoms, their aggravating and alleviating factors, temporality, and response to medications. It is

Table 2
Medications contributing to drug-induced rhinitis

System	Medication	Mechanism of Action
Cardiovascular	Beta-blockers (propranolol) Alpha-blockers (clonidine) Centrally acting antihypertensives (methyldopa, reserpine) Angiotensin converting enzyme inhibitors Vasodilators (hydralazine) Diuretics (hydrochlorothiazide) Niacin	Interferes with normal sympathetic tone that causes vasoconstriction of local vessels, leading to vasodilation and symptoms of nasal congestion
Central Nervous System	Typical or atypical antipsychotics Chlormethiazole Citalopram Psychotropics (risperidone, chlorpromazine, amitriptyline) Gabapentin	Alpha-blocking and beta-blocking properties
Endocrine	Oral contraceptives Estrogens Phosphodiesterase 5 inhibitors (sildenafil, tadalafil, vardenafil)	

Other	Aspirin or nonsteroidal antiinflammatory
	  drugs
	Mycophenolate mofetil
	Penicillamine
	Lamivudine
	Metamucil
	Intraocular or ophthalmic preparations of
	  beta-blockers	

important to assess the environment for the presence of animals, tobacco smoke, pollution, and dust inside the home. It should include all comorbid conditions and medications taken. It is also important to rule out disorders such as granulomatous disease, nasal polyposis, cerebrospinal fluid leak, and malignancies. Even though older patients may be of retirement age, long-term occupational exposures from former careers may still be relevant and should be recorded.

Examination should include the external anatomy, inspecting the tip of the nose, and whether there is static or dynamic valve collapse. Internally, the inferior turbinates, septum, and presence secretions should be assessed. Nasal endoscopy is often useful and should be considered as part of a thorough nasal examination.

Allergy testing is useful to determine atopic status. Other investigations, such as sinus computed tomography (CT) scan or MRI, are indicated when there is a lack of response to medical treatment, when there is suspicion of an underlying cause for the symptoms such as tumors, or for planning sinus or nasal surgery.

TREATMENT
Allergic Rhinitis

Specific treatments include reduction or elimination of allergens from the patient environment, pharmacologic treatment, and immunotherapy. Surgery is reserved for symptoms that are refractory to medical treatments.

Environmental management

Environmental management includes avoidance of exposures to allergens, some of which are present all year round and others which are seasonal. If the patient is allergic to *Dermatophagoides* (dust mites), a bedroom with large windows is preferable (airing it out easily), high beds, washable (uncarpeted) floors, limited dust-accumulating elements, and dust mite covers for pillows and mattresses. If the patient is allergic to pollen, traveling with closed windows and leaving used clothing outside the bedroom during the day should be recommended. For nasal dryness, the use of saline nasal irrigation is useful by helping to clear the mucus and moisten the nasal mucosa.

Pharmacologic treatment

The principal concern with medications in the elderly pertains to the possibility of interactions with other drugs and diseases. The risk of adverse events increases exponentially with the number of drugs used and with concomitant liver or renal impairment. The type of drug used should be related to the clinical symptoms of rhinitis; for example, if the predominant symptom is nasal obstruction, then intranasal corticosteroids should be used. Intranasal corticosteroids and intranasal and/or oral antihistamine drugs constitute first-line therapies.[41] Other medications that can be used include anticholinergics, intranasal chromones, oral decongestants, and leukotriene antagonists.

Intranasal corticosteroids Intranasal corticosteroids are used in upper airway diseases, including allergic and nonallergic rhinitis, and are recommended as first-line treatment regardless of the severity in patients older than 60 years of age.[42,43] They reduce nasal congestion, pruritus, rhinorrhea, eye symptoms, and sneezing.[44] They potentially reduce nasal inflammation and are currently the most effective treatment of allergic rhinitis. However, they have a slow onset of action compared with antihistamines, and a trial of 1 week minimum should be attempted. Side effects such as nasal irritation and bleeding are rare, and septal perforations are an exception. There are no data to suggest an increase in side effects from the use of these drugs in older patients.[45] Mometasone and ciclesonide have minimal bioavailability and, therefore, are the safest options; this characteristic is particularly important in the elderly.[46]

Antihistamines: Antihistamines are widely used for allergic rhinitis, conjunctivitis, and allergic skin diseases in elderly patients. They act by blocking H1 receptors on smooth muscle cells, nerve endings, and glandular cells.

First-generation antihistamines such as chlorpheniramine, diphenhydramine, triprolidine, and hydroxyzine, are associated with marked sedation. Other undesirable side-effects from these medications include anticholinergic effects (dry mouth, blurred vision); cognitive alteration and central nervous system effects (drowsiness and global alteration); cardiovascular effects; and interactions with fluoxetine, cimetidine, macrolides, and ketoconazole. Although these first-generation antihistamines control the symptoms of allergic rhinitis effectively, their side effects limit their usefulness, especially in older patients.

Second-generation H1-receptor antagonists provide excellent, safe, and effective treatment of allergic rhinitis in elderly patients, thanks to a relatively low rate of passage across the blood–brain barrier. This results in much less sedation, and the higher specificity for the H1 receptor decreases anticholinergic and antiserotonergic side effects. Fexofenadine, cetirizine, loratadine, levocetirizine, desloratadine, bilastine, and ebastine are most commonly used in elderly people.[47] Interactions with other drugs are relatively minimal but because they are metabolized by the cytochrome 450 enzyme during their first pass through the liver they are not recommended for patients with significant liver disease.[48] Patients with renal impairment should take lower daily doses of antihistamines such as azelastine, ebastine, desloratadine, and cetirizine because they are excreted by the kidney.[49] They act rapidly and are effective against pruritus, sneezing, rhinorrhea, and ocular symptoms, and their effects can last up to 7 days after ceasing of the medication.

Topical antihistamines (azelastine, levocabastine, and olopatadine) have effects that are comparable to systemic second-generation antihistamines but have the added advantages of a quicker onset of action and of not inducing systemic adverse reactions. Furthermore, if combined with a topical corticosteroid, they may have more than an additive effect on symptoms. However, they generally have to be taken twice daily.

Decongestants Local or systemic decongestants relieve nasal obstruction thanks to their sympathomimetic properties, which is a significant problem in affected patients. However, they do not relieve symptoms such as sneezing, pruritus, and secretions.[50] They act on alpha-adrenergic vessels, producing vasoconstriction.

Oral decongestants, such as pseudoephedrine, may generate many adverse side effects, such as hypertension, palpitations, headache, agitation, tremor, insomnia, dry mucosa, urinary retention, and exacerbation of glaucoma or thyrotoxicosis.[47] Thus, they must be avoided in older patients with multiple comorbid conditions, such as coronary artery disease, diabetes, hypertension, hyperthyroidism, narrow-angle glaucoma, and symptoms of bladder neck obstruction.

The major side effect of topical decongestants is their potential to induce rebound congestion if used for more than 5 consecutive days, which may lead to rhinitis medicamentosa. These should be used only for short-term courses and not as monotherapy.

Antileukotrienes Antileukotrienes are selective and competitive receptor antagonists for the activity of leukotriene D4 and E4. They decrease the inflammatory response in allergic rhinitis and improve nasal and ocular symptoms but are less effective than antihistamines and topical steroids. The combination of antileukotrienes and antihistamines showed a synergistic effect for the treatment of seasonal allergic rhinitis. These medications are particularly useful in asthmatics, where they may have the additional benefit of improving lower airway disease.

Anticholinergics The principle agent used is ipratropium bromide, which blocks muscarinic receptors, leading to a decrease in the parasympathetic function. It is only effective against anterior rhinorrhea. These medications are usually indicated in combination with a topical corticosteroid or with an antihistamine.

Allergen-specific immunotherapy
Allergen-specific immunotherapy is the only disease-modifying treatment for allergic patients. There is no age limit for prescribing immunotherapy in the elderly[51] and advanced age is no longer a contraindication.[52] It should only be considered in patients with clinical nasal symptoms associated with a confirmation of an IgE-mediated reaction to a specific inhalant allergen. There is evidence demonstrating that it is effective in the elderly. It causes a reduction in symptoms, drug consumption, and new sensitization.[53] It also decreases both cutaneous sensitivity and specific IgE levels, leading to improved clinical symptoms.[54] It is contraindicated in patients with uncontrolled asthma or significant cardiovascular diseases, and it should be

administered with caution to patients on beta-blockers or angiotensin-converting enzyme inhibitors[55,56] because of the higher risk of anaphylactic shock.[57] Comorbid conditions and contraindications should be evaluated carefully before an elderly patient is started on immunotherapy. Traditionally, subcutaneous immunotherapy (SCIT) was used; however, a growing trend toward sublingual immunotherapy (SLIT) has been noted, first in Europe, then in North America. Whether SCIT or SLIT is used, there is equal efficacy in treatment; however, the risk of systemic side effects must be taken into account. The incidence of SCIT-induced systemic reactions is 0.1%,[58] whereas SLIT has a better safety profile.[59] Because of this and its ability to be administered at home, the use of SLIT is recommended in the elderly population.[60] In elderly patients, immunotherapy may reduce the use of other medications.

Nonallergic Rhinitis

Idiopathic or vasomotor rhinitis
Anticholinergics work well for rhinorrhea and are the traditional gold standard treatment of this condition. They have not; however, been studied specifically in elderly patients. The US Food and Drug Administration has approved the use of intranasal azelastine, which has antiinflammatory effects and improves rhinorrhea, sneezing, postnasal drip, and congestion.[61]

Gustatory rhinorrhea
Topical ipratropium bromide before ingestion of the trigger food has been shown to be an effective treatment.[62,63] It has few local side effects such as epistaxis and nasal dryness. This drug should, however, be avoided in patients with angle-closure glaucoma or with urinary retention due to benign prostatic hypertrophy.

Atrophic rhinitis
The goal of treatment of atrophic rhinitis is to reduce symptoms, to improve quality of life, and to eliminate secondary bacterial infections, reducing the amount of crusts and the associated odor. Management consists primarily of education regarding nasal hygiene and the use of antibiotics. Continuous and regular nasal hygiene with high-pressure irrigation remains the mainstay of conservative therapy. Moisturizing measures should be accompanied by the removal of the crusts. Systemic antibiotic therapy should be guided by nasal culture results. The antibiotics of preference, taking into account the main pathogens (gram-negative bacteria), are aminoglycosides, rifampicin 600 mg once daily for 12 weeks, and ciprofloxacin 500 to 750 mg twice daily for 8 to 12 weeks.[39,64] In cases of malnutrition or iron, zinc, protein, and vitamin A deficiencies, supplements are recommended.[39]

SURGERY

Surgery is effective for older individuals; however, functional status, comorbidities, and the anesthetic risk of each geriatric patient must be assessed preoperatively to determine if surgery is a suitable option. Nasal reconstruction can be performed to reverse the effects of aging on the nose, including raising the nasal tip, supporting the lateral cartilages and improving aesthetic appereance.[65] These could also help air flow and nasal function. Septoplasty and turbinoplasty have been shown to improve symptoms and reduce medication usage. In addition, quality of life scores in geriatric patients who present with nasal obstruction due to septal deviation and inferior turbinate hypertrophy improve after the surgery.[66] Radiofrequency turbinoplasty is well-tolerated and seems to be effective for treating some nonallergic rhinitis symptoms in elderly patients, including rhinorrhea and nasal obstruction.[67]

CHRONIC RHINOSINUSITIS

Chronic rhinosinusitis (CRS) is a highly prevalent disease and is defined as symptomatic inflammation of the nasal mucosa and paranasal cavities for more than 3 months duration. It is considered the second most frequent chronic condition in the United States, and it is the sixth most common chronic disease in the elderly population.[5] It affects approximately 5% to 15% of the general population, both in Europe and the United States.[68] Studies of CRS in the elderly population are generally limited; however, an increased incidence of polyposis in the elderly has been well-described in the recent literature. A 2011 review of the Korean National Health System data revealed that the incidence of CRS with polyps doubles in patients older than the age of 65 years.[69] Cho and colleagues[70] described that nasal polyps and asthma tended to be more prevalent in elderly patients compared with nonelderly patients, and that CT scan scores of the elderly group were significantly worse than those of the nonelderly group.[71]

For the diagnosis of CRS, subjective criteria are required, including 2 or more symptoms, among which should be nasal obstruction, blockage, or congestion or nasal discharge (anterior or posterior nasal drip); plus or minus facial pain or pressure, or hyposmia, for more than 12 weeks. Additionally, 1 objective finding is required either on nasal endoscopy (nasal polyps and/or mucopurulent discharge and/or oedema or mucosal obstruction in the middle meatus) or a CT scan (mucosal changes within the ostiomeatal complex and/or sinuses).[68]

A recent study showed no differences in clinical presentation between older and younger patients, either in associated cofactors (prevalence of smoking, polyps, asthma, and aspirin sensitivity), quality-of-life instruments, or objective measures of disease severity, including a Lund-MacKay CT scan and Lund-Kennedy endoscopic scoring.[72]

TREATMENT

Most patients with CRS require medical treatment over many years. The goal of treatment is to achieve and maintain clinical control, which is defined as having no symptoms or symptoms that are not very bothersome. Ideally, this is associated with healthy nasal mucosa with minimal topical treatment.[73] The treatment recommendations of European Position Paper on Rhinosinusitis and Nasal Polyposis (EPOS)-2012[68] are based on the evaluation of symptoms using a visual analog scale and endoscopic evaluation.

For CRS without nasal polyps, topical corticosteroids and nasal irrigations with saline solution (level of evidence Ia, recommendation A), and reevaluation in 3 months are recommended. For patients with moderate and severe symptoms, the use of long-term antibiotics can be added. For example, macrolides can be prescribed for 12 weeks, especially in patients with a low or normal total serum IgE (level of evidence Ib, recommendation C). However, caution is advised because drug interactions with macrolides are common (especially with clarithromycin), and adverse cardiac events have been described with azithromycin. In moderate and severe cases with patients who have failed medical management, it is recommended to perform a CT scan of the paranasal sinuses and consider surgical treatment.[68]

For CRS with nasal polyps (CRSwNP), patients with mild disease should receive topical corticosteroids (level of evidence Ia, recommendation A) and nasal irrigations with saline solution (recommendation D) and be reevaluated after 3 months. For patients with moderate symptoms, the additional use of antibiotics like doxycycline should be considered (level of evidence Ib, recommendation A). In the severe group, oral corticosteroids should be prescribed (level of evidence Ia, recommendation A), in the absence of any contraindications. In both moderate and severe patients, it is recommended to perform a CT scan of the paranasal sinuses and consider surgical treatment, if no improvement is seen with medical treatment.[68]

In older patients, because of possible comorbidities and polypharmacy, caution has to be taken with the prescription of medications for CRS. Intranasal corticosteroids and saline solution are quite safe in the elderly population. Broad-spectrum antibiotics, such as third-generation cephalosporins, fluoroquinolones, and clindamycin, can also cause *Clostridium difficile* colitis, which is more common and fatal in the elderly compared with younger adults.[74] Oral steroids must be prescribed with caution because there are significant side effects, many of which are age-dependent (ie, osteoporosis, diabetes, and arterial hypertension).

Surgery

When maximal medical treatment fails, surgery should be considered, regardless of age. Because this is a disease that significantly affects the quality of life but is not life-threatening, the patient's comorbidities and anesthetic risk must be taken into account. If the benefit to the patient outweighs the risk, surgery should be offered. Endoscopic sinus surgery (ESS) in the geriatric population is a safe and effective treatment of CRS refractory to medical therapy.[5,75]

Evidence shows that ESS results are similar in the older and younger patient populations, with a similar degree of improvement on endoscopy scores and quality-of-life measures.[5,72] Ramadan and VanMetre[76] performed a retrospective study comparing complications in ESS in adults (18–64 years old) and older patients (64 years old). They found that older adults had higher overall complication rates but that this was mainly caused by higher rates of revision surgery in the older group. Primary ESS complication rates were similar between the 2 groups. Another study found no differences in complication rate between the 2 groups.[5]

SUMMARY

The geriatric population has increased worldwide, and sinonasal disorders are frequent in this population. When untreated, they can significantly affect patients' quality of life and may exacerbate respiratory diseases. With advancing age, there are several changes in both nasal physiology and anatomy, as well as in the immune system; these changes can influence the onset of rhinitis and rhinosinusitis symptoms in older adults.

The evaluation of the elderly patient should include a full history of the symptoms with a careful assessment of comorbidities; potential drug interactions should be considered before prescribing any pharmacologic therapy. A correct diagnosis of the rhinitis subtype is essential to improve the success of therapy and improve quality of life.

Surgery can be considered in this group provided the patient's comorbidities and anesthetic risk have been taken into account. In patients in whom the benefits outweigh the risks, surgery should be offered as a management option.

REFERENCES

1. Statistics Canada. Table 051-001-estimates of population by age group and sex for July 1, Canada, provinces and territories, CANSIM. Ottawa (Canada): Statistics Canada; 2010.

2. Ortman JM, Velkoff VA, Hogan H. An aging nation: the older population in the United States. Washington, DC: US Census Bureau; 2014.
3. Staecker H. Introduction to geriatric otolaryngology. 1st edition. New York: Tailor & Francis Group; 2006.
4. Statistics Canada. Life expectancy, at birth and at age 65, by sex and by province and territory 2012. Available at: www.statcan.gc.ca/daily-quotidien/160519/dq160519c-eng.htm. Accessed May 31, 2012.
5. Jiang RS, Hsu CY. Endoscopic sinus surgery for the treatment of chronic sinusitis in geriatric patients. Ear Nose Throat J 2001;80(4):230–2.
6. Piccirillo JF, Merritt MG Jr, Richards ML. Psychometric and clinimetric validity of the 20-item sino-nasal outcome test (SNOT-20). Otolaryngol Head Neck Surg 2002;126(1):41–7.
7. DelGaudio JM, Panella NJ. Presbynasalis. Int Forum Allergy Rhinol 2016;6(10):1083–7.
8. Edelstein DR. Aging of the normal nose in adults. Laryngoscope 1996;106(9 Pt 2):1–25.
9. Loftus PA, Wise SK, Nieto D, et al. Intranasal volume increases with age: computed tomography volumetric analysis in adults. Laryngoscope 2016;126(10):2212–5.
10. Nappi C, Di Spiezio Sardo A, Guerra G, et al. Functional and morphologic evaluation of the nasal mucosa before and after hormone therapy in postmenopausal women with nasal symptoms. Fertil Steril 2003;80(3):669–71.
11. Ho JC, Chan KN, Hu WH, et al. The effect of aging on nasal mucociliary clearance, beat frequency, and ultrastructure of respiratory cilia. Am J Respir Crit Care Med 2001;163(4):983–8.
12. Busse PJ, Mathur SK. Age-related changes in immune function: effect on airway inflammation. J Allergy Clin Immunol 2010;126(4):690–9 [quiz: 700–91].
13. Bende M. Blood flow with 133Xe in human nasal mucosa in relation to age, sex and body position. Acta Otolaryngol 1983;96(1–2):175–9.
14. Salvioli S, Monti D, Lanzarini C, et al. Immune system, cell senescence, aging and longevity–inflamm-aging reappraised. Curr Pharm Des 2013;19(9):1675–9.
15. Hinojosa E, Boyd AR, Orihuela CJ. Age-associated inflammation and toll-like receptor dysfunction prime the lungs for pneumococcal pneumonia. J Infect Dis 2009;200(4):546–54.
16. Agarwal S, Busse PJ. Innate and adaptive immunosenescence. Ann Allergy Asthma Immunol 2010;104(3):183–90 [quiz: 190–2, 210].
17. Paik SI, Lehman MN, Seiden AM, et al. Human olfactory biopsy. The influence of age and receptor distribution. Arch Otolaryngol Head Neck Surg 1992;118(7):731–8.
18. Schriever VA, Reither N, Gerber J, et al. Olfactory bulb volume in smokers. Exp Brain Res 2013;225(2):153–7.
19. Murphy C, Schubert CR, Cruickshanks KJ, et al. Prevalence of olfactory impairment in older adults. JAMA 2002;288(18):2307–12.
20. Seiberling KA, Conley DB. Aging and olfactory and taste function. Otolaryngol Clin North Am 2004;37(6):1209–28, vii.
21. Rossi S, Ulivelli M. The olfactory side of Parkinson disease: relevance for clinical practice. Neurology 2015;85(15):1266–7.
22. Doty RL. Olfactory dysfunction in Parkinson disease. Nat Rev Neurol 2012;8(6):329–39.
23. Zucco GM, Zaglis D, Wambsganss CS. Olfactory deficits in elderly subjects and Parkinson patients. Percept Mot Skills 1991;73(3 Pt 1):895–8.

24. Apter AJ, Mott AE, Frank ME, et al. Allergic rhinitis and olfactory loss. Ann Allergy Asthma Immunol 1995;75(4):311–6.
25. Sivam A, Jeswani S, Reder L, et al. Olfactory cleft inflammation is present in seasonal allergic rhinitis and is reduced with intranasal steroids. Am J Rhinol Allergy 2010;24(4):286–90.
26. Enright PL, Kronmal RA, Higgins MW, et al. Prevalence and correlates of respiratory symptoms and disease in the elderly. Cardiovascular Health Study. Chest 1994;106(3):827–34.
27. Shargorodsky J, Garcia-Esquinas E, Galan I, et al. Allergic sensitization, rhinitis and tobacco smoke exposure in US adults. PLoS One 2015;10(7):e0131957.
28. Rawle FC, Burr ML, Platts-Mills TA. Long-term falls in antibodies to dust mite and pollen allergens in patients with asthma or hay fever. Clin Allergy 1983;13(5): 409–17.
29. Meltzer EO. The prevalence and medical and economic impact of allergic rhinitis in the United States. J Allergy Clin Immunol 1997;99(6 Pt 2):S805–28.
30. Simola M, Holopainene E, Malmberg H. Changes in skin and nasal sensitivity to allergens and the course of rhinitis; a long-term follow-up study. Ann Allergy Asthma Immunol 1999;82(2):152–6.
31. Pinto JM, Jeswani S. Rhinitis in the geriatric population. Allergy Asthma Clin Immunol 2010;6(1):10.
32. Hakansson K, von Buchwald C, Thomsen SF, et al. Nonallergic rhinitis and its association with smoking and lower airway disease: a general population study. Am J Rhinol Allergy 2011;25(1):25–9.
33. Lal D, Corey JP. Vasomotor rhinitis update. Curr Opin Otolaryngol Head Neck Surg 2004;12(3):243–7.
34. Baptist AP, Nyenhuis S. Rhinitis in the elderly. Immunol Allergy Clin North Am 2016;36(2):343–57.
35. Hansen I, Klimek L, Mosges R, et al. Mediators of inflammation in the early and the late phase of allergic rhinitis. Curr Opin Allergy Clin Immunol 2004;4(3): 159–63.
36. Sahin Yilmaz AA, Corey JP. Rhinitis in the elderly. Curr Allergy Asthma Rep 2006; 6(2):125–31.
37. Di Lorenzo G, Leto-Barone MS, La Piana S, et al. Clinical course of rhinitis and changes in vivo and in vitro of allergic parameters in elderly patients: a long-term follow-up study. Clin Exp Med 2013;13(1):67–73.
38. Bousquet J, Khaltaev N, Cruz AA, et al. Allergic rhinitis and its impact on asthma (ARIA) 2008 update (in collaboration with the World Health Organization, GA(2) LEN and AllerGen). Allergy 2008;63(Suppl 86):8–160.
39. Dutt SN, Kameswaran M. The aetiology and management of atrophic rhinitis. J Laryngol Otol 2005;119(11):843–52.
40. Kaufman DW, Kelly JP, Rosenberg L, et al. Recent patterns of medication use in the ambulatory adult population of the United States: the Slone survey. JAMA 2002;287(3):337–44.
41. Brozek JL, Bousquet J, Agache I, et al. Allergic rhinitis and its impact on asthma (ARIA) guidelines-2016 revision. J Allergy Clin Immunol 2017;140:950–8.
42. Wallace DV, Dykewicz MS, Bernstein DI, et al. The diagnosis and management of rhinitis: an updated practice parameter. J Allergy Clin Immunol 2008; 122(2 Suppl):S1–84.
43. Can D, Tanac R, Demir E, et al. Is the usage of intranasal glucocorticosteroids alone in allergic rhinitis sufficient? Allergy Asthma Proc 2006;27(3):248–53.

44. Penagos M, Compalati E, Tarantini F, et al. Efficacy of mometasone furoate nasal spray in the treatment of allergic rhinitis. Meta-analysis of randomized, double-blind, placebo-controlled, clinical trials. Allergy 2008;63(10):1280–91.

45. Bozek A. Pharmacological management of allergic rhinitis in the elderly. Drugs Aging 2017;34(1):21–8.

46. Bielory L, Blaiss M, Fineman SM, et al. Concerns about intranasal corticosteroids for over-the-counter use: position statement of the Joint Task Force for the American Academy of Allergy, Asthma and Immunology and the American College of Allergy, Asthma and Immunology. Ann Allergy Asthma Immunol 2006;96(4): 514–25.

47. Hansen J, Klimek L, Hormann K. Pharmacological management of allergic rhinitis in the elderly: safety issues with oral antihistamines. Drugs Aging 2005;22(4): 289–96.

48. Simons FE. The antiallergic effects of antihistamines (H1-receptor antagonists). J Allergy Clin Immunol 1992;90(4 Pt 2):705–15.

49. Kaliner MA. H1-antihistamines in the elderly. Clin Allergy Immunol 2002;17: 465–81.

50. Horak F, Zieglmayer P, Zieglmayer R, et al. A placebo-controlled study of the nasal decongestant effect of phenylephrine and pseudoephedrine in the Vienna Challenge Chamber. Ann Allergy Asthma Immunol 2009;102(2):116–20.

51. Zuberbier T, Bachert C, Bousquet PJ, et al. GA(2) LEN/EAACI pocket guide for allergen-specific immunotherapy for allergic rhinitis and asthma. Allergy 2010; 65(12):1525–30.

52. Pitsios C, Demoly P, Bilo MB, et al. Clinical contraindications to allergen immunotherapy: an EAACI position paper. Allergy 2015;70(8):897–909.

53. Marogna M, Bruno ME, Massolo A, et al. Sublingual immunotherapy for allergic respiratory disease in elderly patients: a retrospective study. Eur Ann Allergy Clin Immunol 2008;40(1):22–9.

54. Armentia A, Fernandez A, Tapias JA, et al. Immunotherapy with allergenic extracts in geriatric patients: evaluation of effectiveness and safety. Allergol Immunopathol (Madr) 1993;21(5):193–6.

55. Jutel M, Kosowska A, Smolinska S. Allergen Immunotherapy: past, present, and future. Allergy Asthma Immunol Res 2016;8(3):191–7.

56. Cox L, Nelson H, Lockey R, et al. Allergen immunotherapy: a practice parameter third update. J Allergy Clin Immunol 2011;127(1 Suppl):S1–55.

57. Jutel M, Agache I, Bonini S, et al. International consensus on allergen immunotherapy II: mechanisms, standardization, and pharmacoeconomics. J Allergy Clin Immunol 2016;137(2):358–68.

58. Epstein TG, Liss GM, Murphy-Berendts K, et al. Immediate and delayed-onset systemic reactions after subcutaneous immunotherapy injections: ACAAI/AAAAI surveillance study of subcutaneous immunotherapy: year 2. Ann Allergy Asthma Immunol 2011;107(5):426–31.e1.

59. Canonica GW, Bousquet J, Casale T, et al. Sub-lingual immunotherapy: World Allergy Organization position paper 2009. Allergy 2009;64(Suppl 91):1–59.

60. Hur GY, Lee JH, Park HS. Allergen immunotherapy for the treatment of respiratory allergies in the elderly. Curr Opin Allergy Clin Immunol 2017;17(4):304–8.

61. Banov CH, Lieberman P, Vasomotor Rhinitis Study Groups. Efficacy of azelastine nasal spray in the treatment of vasomotor (perennial nonallergic) rhinitis. Ann Allergy Asthma Immunol 2001;86(1):28–35.

62. Waibel KH, Chang C. Prevalence and food avoidance behaviors for gustatory rhinitis. Ann Allergy Asthma Immunol 2008;100(3):200–5.

63. Raphael G, Raphael MH, Kaliner M. Gustatory rhinitis: a syndrome of food-induced rhinorrhea. J Allergy Clin Immunol 1989;83(1):110–5.
64. Moore EJ, Kern EB. Atrophic rhinitis: a review of 242 cases. Am J Rhinol 2001; 15(6):355–61.
65. Hong HR, Kim SH, Kim JH, et al. Aesthetic motivation of geriatric rhinoplasty the surgical outcome. J Craniofac Surg 2015;26(6):1936–9.
66. Busaba NY, Hossain M. Clinical outcomes of septoplasty and inferior turbinate reduction in the geriatric veterans' population. Am J Rhinol 2004;18(6):343–7.
67. Yu MS, Kang SH, Kim BH, et al. Radiofrequency turbinoplasty for nonallergic rhinitis in geriatric patients. Am J Rhinol Allergy 2015;29(5):e134–137.
68. Fokkens WJ, Lund VJ, Mullol J, et al. European position paper on rhinosinusitis and nasal polyps 2012. Rhinol Suppl 2012;23. 3 p preceding table of contents, 1–298.
69. Kim YS, Kim NH, Seong SY, et al. Prevalence and risk factors of chronic rhinosinusitis in Korea. Am J Rhinol Allergy 2011;25(3):117–21.
70. Cho SH, Kim DW, Lee SH, et al. Age-related increased prevalence of asthma and nasal polyps in chronic rhinosinusitis and its association with altered IL-6 trans-signaling. Am J Respir Cell Mol Biol 2015;53(5):601–6.
71. Cho SH, Hong SJ, Han B, et al. Age-related differences in the pathogenesis of chronic rhinosinusitis. J Allergy Clin Immunol 2012;129(3):858–60.e2.
72. Reh DD, Mace J, Robinson JL, et al. Impact of age on presentation of chronic rhinosinusitis and outcomes of endoscopic sinus surgery. Am J Rhinol 2007;21(2): 207–13.
73. Bhattacharyya N, Orlandi RR, Grebner J, et al. Cost burden of chronic rhinosinusitis: a claims-based study. Otolaryngol Head Neck Surg 2011;144(3):440–5.
74. Kee VR. Clostridium difficile infection in older adults: a review and update on its management. Am J Geriatr Pharmacother 2012;10(1):14–24.
75. Colclasure JC, Gross CW, Kountakis SE. Endoscopic sinus surgery in patients older than sixty. Otolaryngol Head Neck Surg 2004;131(6):946–9.
76. Ramadan HH, VanMetre R. Endoscopic sinus surgery in geriatric population. Am J Rhinol 2004;18(2):125–7.

Head and Neck Cancer in the Elderly

Frailty, Shared Decisions, and Avoidance of Low Value Care

Leila J. Mady, MD, PhD, MPH[a], Marci L. Nilsen, PhD, RN[b],
Jonas T. Johnson, MD[a,c,d,e],*

KEYWORDS

- Head and neck cancer • Older adult oncology • Frailty • Shared decision making
- Patient-centered care • Supportive and palliative care

KEY POINTS

- Head and neck cancer is a disease of older adults, with an estimated 61% of patients ages 65 and older by the year 2030.
- Even with treatment advancements, recurrent/metastatic head and neck squamous cell carcinoma remains a lethal disease with median overall survival of less than 12 months.
- It is imperative to distinguish fit individuals, who may tolerate multimodality therapy, from frail patients, who may benefit from prehabilitation or palliative and supportive services.
- Chemotherapy, radiation, and targeted molecular agents have limited efficacy when used for the palliation of symptoms in advanced disease.
- Shared decision making considers evidence-based best practices in the context of a patient's goals and values and forms the foundation of end-of-life considerations in geriatric oncology.

The authors have nothing to disclose.
[a] Department of Otolaryngology, University of Pittsburgh, School of Medicine, Eye and Ear Institute, Suite 500, 203 Lothrop Street, Pittsburgh, PA 15213, USA; [b] Department of Acute and Tertiary Care, University of Pittsburgh, School of Nursing, 318A Victoria Building, 3500 Victoria Street, Pittsburgh, PA 15261, USA; [c] Department of Radiation Oncology, University of Pittsburgh, School of Medicine, 5230 Centre Avenue, Pittsburgh, PA 15232, USA; [d] Department of Oral and Maxillofacial Surgery, University of Pittsburgh, School of Dental Medicine, 3501 Terrace Street, Pittsburgh, PA 15261, USA; [e] Department of Communication Science and Disorders, University of Pittsburgh, School of Health and Rehabilitation Sciences, Forbes Tower, 3600 Atwood Street, Pittsburgh, PA 15260, USA
* Corresponding author. Eye and Ear Institute, Suite 500, 203 Lothrop Street, Pittsburgh, PA 15213.
E-mail address: johnsonjt@upmc.edu

Clin Geriatr Med 34 (2018) 233–244
https://doi.org/10.1016/j.cger.2018.01.003
0749-0690/18/© 2018 Elsevier Inc. All rights reserved.

INTRODUCTION

Head and neck cancer (HNC) refers to a diverse group of histopathologic malignancies that can originate in the upper aerodigestive tract. More than 90% are squamous cell carcinomas that arise from the mucosal surfaces of the oral cavity, oropharynx, and larynx.[1] In the setting of early disease (stages I–II), there is an 80% cure rate with single-modality therapy, either surgery or radiotherapy.[2,3] A majority of patients (>60%) with head and neck squamous cell carcinoma (HNSCC), however, present with locoregionally advanced disease (stages III and IVA/B) and metastatic tumors (stage IVC).[2,4] Despite multimodality therapy, more than half of patients with locally advanced HNSSC develop recurrences and 30% are at risk of distant metastases.[5,6]

Survival Rates

Survival rates have demonstrated only marginal improvements over the past 30 years, with 5-year overall survival rates reported between 40% and 60%.[7] The growing incidence of human papillomavirus–associated oropharyngeal HNSCC as well as advances in multimodality therapy, including targeted therapy, intensity-modulated radiotherapy, and minimally invasive surgery, have contributed to observed improvements in prognosis.[8,9] Emerging immunotherapeutic agents are also promising developments currently undergoing clinical testing.[3,10] Despite these advancements, recurrent or metastatic HNSSC remains a lethal disease with median overall survival of less than 12 months.[11]

Epidemiologic Trends

The theory of "epidemiologic transition" describes the shift from infectious to degenerative and chronic diseases as the primary causes of morbidity and mortality, particularly in developed countries.[12] The concept illustrates the evolution of neoplastic disease in the setting of increasing life expectancy. Between 1980 and 2000, adults ages 65 and older in the United States increased by 10 million, with a projected doubling in growth to 72 million by 2030.[13] Given advanced age is the most significant risk factor for cancer overall, increases in age-related malignancy rates and survivors will challenge current treatment paradigms.[13,14] Between 2010 and 2030, a 67% increase in overall cancer incidence is projected for patients ages 65 and older.[13] HNSCC demonstrates comparable epidemiologic trends. Despite the increasing proportion of human papillomavirus–positive oropharyngeal cancers, which characteristically affect younger patients, HNC remains a disease of older adults.[15] By 2030, an estimated 61% of HNC patients will be ages 65 and older.[13]

Older patients have been historically underrepresented or excluded from clinical trials, which define standards of care, with only 3.4% of current studies globally involving patients older than 65 years.[15,16] In a meta-analysis of HNC chemotherapy, only 4% of patients across 93 clinical trials were older than 70 years.[17] In the absence of high-level evidence to drive treatment models, a multidisciplinary approach to understand the goals of elderly patients and their caregivers is paramount.

Treatment at the End of Life

Despite the introduction of the Medicare hospice benefit in 1983, care for patients at the end of life comprises more than 25% of Medicare expenditures. Between 1978 and 2006, multiple hospitalizations in the last few months of life and the use of intensive/coronary care units increased among Medicare patients ages 65 and older.[18] The is consistent with reported trends in increased aggressiveness of inpatient and cancer care near the end of life.[19] More than 30% of elderly Americans undergo surgery in the last year of life, with a majority of interventions occurring in the month before death.[20] In a survey of Americans older than 60 years, 75% reported they would not elect surgery if they knew they would live less than 1 year with severe impairment.[21]

From a systems approach, overuse in health care is defined as services in which potential harms exceed benefits.[22] Eliminating overuse is 1 approach to improving value in cancer care. From a patient-centered perspective, treatment modalities that fail to meet the goals of the patient can be defined as low-value care. To approach end-of-life considerations in geriatric oncology, clinical team members must be able to guide patients and caregivers to make decisions that reflect their goals and values.

HOW TO APPROACH THE OLDER ADULT WITH HEAD AND NECK CANCER
Identifying the Frail Patient

Chronologic age alone is not a consistent predictor of life expectancy, treatment-related toxicity, or perioperative risk.[3,23] Because senescence is a heterogenous process, it is imperative to identify those who are fit, who may tolerate standard-of-care therapy, and those who are frail, who may benefit from prehabilitation or palliative intervention. Frailty is a syndrome—distinct from age, comorbidity, or disability alone—which describes decreased physiologic reserve and resistance to stressors. Being frail leaves patients more vulnerable to poor health outcomes, including falls, worsening mobility and activities of daily living disability, hospitalizations, and death.[24]

Although there is no consensus on how to measure frailty, a comprehensive assessment should include physical performance (gait speed and mobility), nutritional status, mental health, and cognition.[25] The Fried frailty phenotype assessment and the Rockwood and Minitski frailty index are 2 of the most commonly used measurements in clinical practice, although there are multiple indices available. Readers are directed to a recent review by Dent and colleagues[26] as well as David Eibling's article, "Frailty and Polypharmacy in Older Patients with Otolaryngologic Diseases," in this issue for further discussion on the topic.

Although traditional oncologic measures (Karnofsky Performance scale[27] and Eastern Cooperative Oncology Group Performance Status[28]) have been used to assess functional status, these instruments have not been validated in the elderly, are subjective, and do not sufficiently capture information regarding comorbidities and physiologic impairment.[3] The comprehensive geriatric assessment (CGA) is a multidisciplinary diagnostic and treatment approach to identify the medical, psychosocial, and functional limitations of older adults with the goal of coordinating care to maximize overall health.[29,30] Geriatric assessment in oncology has been shown to predict morbidity and mortality, modify initial treatment plans, and outperform traditional oncologic measures of performance status in determining "level of fitness."[31,32]

Despite the plethora of literature confirming the utility of CGA, its execution in practice is time intensive and requires trained personnel with geriatric expertise. In response, many geriatric screening tools have been developed including but not limited to the G8 (an 8-question screening questionnaire),[33] abbreviated CGA (aCGA),[34] Groningen Frailty Indicator,[35] and Vulnerable Elders Survey 13.[36] Of these, only the G8 and aCGA were specifically established to assess frailty in the older adult with cancer. Among patients with locoregionally advanced HNSCC, the G8 was able to predict specific cancer-related outcomes, patients with abnormal baseline G8 scores had worse postoperative outcomes, and vulnerable patients identified by G8 screening had lower radiotherapy completion rates among those undergoing radiation therapy

(RT) or chemoradiation therapy (CRT).[37–39] Screening tools are not intended to replace more thorough geriatric assessment; rather, they serve to recognize patients in need of further evaluation. Identification of select geriatric patients who may benefit from more aggressive therapy remains among the most significant challenges in clinical practice.

Guidelines to Approach Decision Making in Older Adults

According to the 2017 National Comprehensive Cancer Network Clinical Practice Guidelines in Oncology, the approach to decision making in older adults should begin with the question, "Is the patient at moderate or high risk of dying or suffering from cancer considering his or her overall life expectancy?"[40] Life expectancy calculators are available at www.eprognosis.com, which may be used to estimate anticipated life expectancy independent of malignancy. These calculators serve as an adjunct to clinical judgment to determine reasonable estimates of whether cancer will shorten an individual's life expectancy or contribute to cancer-related symptoms during the patient's anticipated life span. Histograms for age-specific life expectancy by gender have also been developed.[41] Assessment of comorbidities and functional impairments may be used to estimate an individual's life expectancy relative to age-matched and gender-matched peers. For example, congestive heart failure, end-stage renal disease, oxygen-dependent chronic obstructive lung disease, and severe functional dependencies in activities of daily living place an older individual below the average life expectancy for that individual's age.[41–43] Early on in the decision-making process, symptom management, palliative care, and social support services should be offered as clinically indicated.

Determination of a patient's competence is one element in obtaining informed consent. Evaluation of competence allows providers to respect patient autonomy while protecting vulnerable populations with cognitive or psychiatric impairment.[44] After this determination of decision-making capacity (or in the event of incompetence, identification of a substitute decision maker), the treatment team must assess a patient's goals and values regarding the management of the cancer. Clinicians have an ethical duty and responsibility to engage patients in shared decision making, which is a central component of patient-centered care.[45] The older patient with HNSCC, particularly in the setting of advanced disease, faces myriad choices regarding treatment options. Often, treatment-related sequelae, including disfigurement and dysfunction, may persist or even progress long after therapy is completed. By sharing in the decision-making process, patients can aid the treatment team in identifying interventions that constitute low-value care.

THERAPEUTIC OPTIONS AND CONSIDERATIONS
Current Treatment Paradigms

In primary early-stage disease, patients may be treated with either surgery or RT. Close routine surveillance is necessary to identify potential recurrences or detect second primary tumors. A majority (>90%) of recurrences are observed within 3 years of initial therapy.[46,47] Locoregionally advanced disease requires combined-modality approaches (surgery, RT, and/or chemotherapy) to optimize tumor control. Nonetheless, advanced HNSCC is associated with a high incidence of local recurrence and distant metastases and more than half these patients relapse despite curative-intent treatment.[5,6] There is a small chance in limited cases for successful salvage treatment with either surgery or (re-)irradiation.[11] For most patients, however, recurrent or metastatic disease is a devastating diagnosis with expected survival of less than a year. Chemotherapy, radiation, and targeted molecular agents have limited efficacy when used for the palliation of symptoms in these patients.[48] In a multi-institutional study of chemotherapy use in end-stage cancer, palliative chemotherapy worsened quality of life for patients with good performance status and added no benefit in quality of life for patients with moderate or poor performance status.[49] In these patients, the goal is to decrease symptom burden and improve quality of life through comprehensive palliative and supportive care.

Supportive Care

Each treatment option, even when used for palliation, presents distinct challenges in the elderly. Mechanical airway obstruction, nonhealing wounds, dehydration, failure to thrive, and life-threatening hemorrhage are just some of the issues that may necessitate inpatient hospitalization. Older age is strongly predictive of treatment-related toxicities, including aspiration pneumonia, dysphagia, and gastrostomy tube dependence.[50,51] There are also increased risks in the elderly from competing noncancer causes of mortality, concomitant comorbidities, and altered age-related drug metabolism.[23] These factors may deter treatment plans or even deteriorate a patient's quality of life at the end of life.

There are struggles related to the diagnosis of HNC beyond the associated short-term and long-term consequences of treatment. Physical health issues, including fatigue, sarcopenia, and cachexia, are all compounded with age-related physiologic and metabolic changes.[52,53] Sarcopenia has been associated with decreased locoregional control and disease-specific survival in RT-treated or CRT-treated HNSCC.[54] Disturbances of neurocognitive and psychosocial function are also nontrivial concerns. In a systematic review of depression among HNC patients, rates up to 40% at diagnosis, 52% during treatment, and 45% at 6 months posttreatment were reported.[55] Depression may be associated with anxiety and body image disturbance and can influence treatment adherence, quality of life, and survival.[56] These distresses are real concerns that must be addressed because HNC patients have increased suicide risk compared with the general population and with patients with other cancers.[57]

Palliative care focuses on establishing goals of care, pain and symptom management, and psychosocial and spiritual support. Palliative care should begin at the time of diagnosis and be delivered alongside anticancer, life-prolonging therapies. Palliative care takes on an even greater role and becomes the center of care as disease-directed, life-prolonging therapies become no longer clinically warranted or desired.[21,58] Several studies have demonstrated superior efficacy in quality of life, neurocognition, symptom control, caregiver burden, and survival when palliative care is initiated early in the disease course.[59,60] Early palliation also provides an invaluable contribution in an area where clinicians generally struggle—communicating prognosis. In a randomized trial of patients with terminal cancer, 31.7% of patients believed their cancer was curable. In this study, patients who received early palliative care had improved understanding of their prognosis and were less likely to receive cytotoxic therapy near the end of life.[61] Despite the known benefits of providing early support services, integrating palliative care into a multidisciplinary care model of HNC requires continued, open dialogue between surgeons, medical and radiation oncologists, dentists, speech-language pathologists, dieticians, rehabilitation therapists, and palliative care specialists.

SHARED DECISION MAKING
Implementation

In the management of HNC, treatment plans may be complex and challenging to comprehend. Shared decision making is a collaborative effort that empowers patients and their providers to make treatment-related decisions together, considering evidence-based best practices in the context of a patient's goals and values. The Agency for Healthcare Research and Quality SHARE Approach outlines a 5-step model for shared decision making (**Table 1**).[62]

Through an invitation to join in the decision-making process, patients can become active participants in their oncologic care. To help patients make informed decisions, treatment options must be explained in an objective, honest, and compassionate manner. Decision aids, which are evidence-based tools designed to help patients deliberate health care options, may be useful prior, during, or after a clinical encounter.[63] Although research strongly demonstrates that patients prefer participation in medical choices, a substantial proportion may still delegate final treatment decisions to their provider.[64] It has been reported that despite similar health outcomes, cancer survivors who preferred physician control over decisions had more trust in their physician.[65]

Decisional Regret

It is critical to explain management options in the context of prognosis and treatment-related toxicities. In a systematic review of decisional regret, risk factors most consistently associated with regret involved the decision-making process and treatment-related issues, in particular posttreatment complications or adverse outcomes.[66] Decisional regret seems to be a general phenomenon, unrelated to specific demographics or populations. Over time, decisional regret may increase, particularly if patient values are not elucidated beforehand. In a survey of 1729 oropharyngeal cancer survivors, 61% reported some degree of regret regarding their treatment choice, of which one-quarter expressed "moderate to strong" regret. In this cohort, symptom burden was the strongest driver of decisional regret with difficulty swallowing followed by feeling sad and pain.[67]

As therapeutic alternatives are evaluated vis-à-vis patient preferences and goals, clinicians must be cognizant of biases in prognostication and perceptions of treatment-related outcomes. Review of physicians' abilities to precisely predict survival demonstrates only a 10% to 30% accuracy rate, with overestimation of survival by a factor of 2 to 5. The longer a provider is involved in the care of a patient, the more likely that provider is to overestimate predictions.[68,69] Discordance between physicians and patients has also been reported regarding perceived attitudes of quality of life after HNC treatment.[70–72] Providers tend to underestimate the severity of pain with treatment, yet survivors may be more willing to accept greater pain intensity in exchange for the potential of being cured.[70] In a study comparing quality-of-life considerations after laryngectomy, physicians deemed communication impairment and self-image/self-esteem as most important whereas patients identified physical

Table 1 The SHARE approach	
S	Seek patients' participation
H	Help patients explore and compare treatment options
A	Assess patients' values and preferences
R	Reach a decision with patients
E	Evaluate patients' decisions

Adapted with permission from Agency for Healthcare Research and Quality. Originally available at: http://www.ahrq.gov/professionals/education/curriculumtools/shareddecisionmaking/index.html

sequelae of surgery and disruption of social activities as most significant.[71] In another study, 46% of health care providers assumed laryngectomy patients would be willing to compromise survival in exchange for voice preservation or preoperative qualify of life when actually only 20% of patients expressed this preference.[72]

The importance of exploring a patient's values and goals through shared decision making cannot be overemphasized. Even in primary early-stage disease, treatment decisions must be assessed apropos patient goals. As discussed previously, curative-intent therapy is often associated with persistent treatment-related effects, which may limit a patient's function, autonomy, and quality of life. In the setting of pre-treatment functional disability and frailty, the sequelae of surgery, chemotherapy, or radiation may be more harmful if a poor or unacceptable functional status results post-treatment—even if oncologic cure or prolonged life is achieved. Standard-of-care therapy may be considered for advanced disease if the challenges associated with multimodality treatment, related side effects, and risk of recurrence or treatment failure are accepted and in line with patient values. When patients indicate goals that are unachievable, however, it is health care providers' responsibility to guide patients toward early comprehensive palliative and support services.

CLINICAL VIGNETTE

A 73-year-old man presented to clinic with recurrent HNSCC of the oral cavity, for which he underwent treatment of his disease 9 months prior. His medical history was significant for polypharmacy and numerous comorbidities, including heart disease, chronic obstructive pulmonary disease related to a 50-pack year tobacco history, and dialysis-dependent chronic kidney disease. On examination, he appeared malnourished, corroborating his history of a 70-pound unintentional weight loss. He described pain along the anterior floor of the mouth, corresponding to findings on imaging (**Fig. 1**).

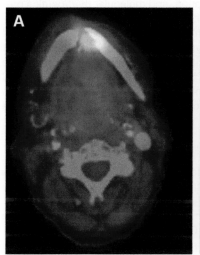
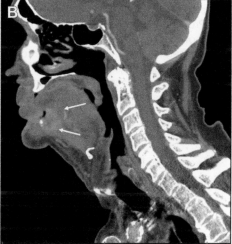

Fig. 1. (*A*) Axial PET/CT image of the neck shows increased FDG avidity associated with the anterior floor of the mouth and some ill-defined tissue. (*B*) Sagittal CT image of the neck with contrast shows a 1.1-cm × 2.1-cm × 2.1-cm ill-defined mass with central necrosis (*arrows*). The mass abuts the genioglossus and geniohyoid muscles and is associated with bony destruction of the mandible extending 3.6 cm in length.

The poor prognosis associated with his disease and salvage options were discussed. Aggressive surgical resection would be necessary in addition to microvascular reconstruction and tracheostomy and gastrostomy tube placement. Using the Best Case/Worst Case model of communication,[73] the surgeon explained that in the best case scenario the patient would endure a protracted recovery course in a skilled cared facility; in the worst case scenario, the patient would die in the hospital without returning home.

To operationalize identification of the frail, the University of Pittsburgh Medical Center has implemented a previously validated screening tool, the Risk Analysis Index,[74] across all surgical services. The initiative aims to create a "surgical pause" prior to the operating room. This pause allows a frail patient to undergo comprehensive multidisciplinary evaluation in the Center for Presurgical Care, where prehabilitation, medical optimization, and consideration of alternatives to surgery may take place. The patient demonstrated significant frailty by this screening method and was referred to the Center for Presurgical Care, where the patient expressed his strong interest to proceed with surgery. Further clarification of his treatment goals revealed his desires to "get healthy again," "get back to life after surgery," and "go back home." In fact, the patient described that it would "kill him" if he could not return home. The discrepancy between his stated goal to return home and his request for surgery elicited from further evaluation became a significant turning point in the clinical team's discussions regarding appropriate therapeutic options. The patient did not undergo further disease-directed therapy and was referred to palliative care.

SUMMARY

The clinical vignette illustrates key issues in the management of geriatric HNC patients. Recurrent and metastatic HNSCC is a lethal disease with median overall survival of less than 12 months. Within this vulnerable population, it is imperative to distinguish those who are fit from those who are frail, who may be unable to tolerate standard-of-care therapy. Chemotherapy, radiation, and molecular therapeutics present distinct challenges in the elderly, with limited efficacy in the palliation of symptoms. Providers have an obligation to inform patients of the true benefits and burdens of these treatments, including the physical and psychosocial sequelae that can be devastating to quality of life. Shared decision making and early comprehensive palliative and support services are at the crux of the approach to older adults with HNC and must be put into action at the time of diagnosis. In doing so, low-value care, which fails to meet the goals of patients and their caregivers at the end-of-life, may be avoided.

REFERENCES

1. Vigneswaran N, Williams MD. Epidemiologic trends in head and neck cancer and aids in diagnosis. Oral Maxillofac Surg Clin North Am 2014;26(2): 123–41.
2. Pulte D, Brenner H. Changes in survival in head and neck cancers in the late 20th and early 21st century: a period analysis. Oncologist 2010;15(9):994–1001.
3. Szturz P, Vermorken JB. Treatment of elderly patients with squamous cell carcinoma of the head and neck. Front Oncol 2016;6:199.
4. Argiris A, Karamouzis MV, Raben D, et al. Head and neck cancer. Lancet 2008; 371(9625):1695–709.
5. Coatesworth AP, Tsikoudas A, MacLennan K. The cause of death in patients with head and neck squamous cell carcinoma. J Laryngol Otol 2002;116(4):269–71.

6. Marur S, Forastiere AA. Head and neck cancer: changing epidemiology, diagnosis, and treatment. Mayo Clin Proc 2008;83(4):489–501.

7. Siegel RL, Miller KD, Jemal A. Cancer statistics, 2015. CA Cancer J Clin 2015; 65(1):5–29.

8. Argiris A, Harrington KJ, Tahara M, et al. Evidence-based treatment options in recurrent and/or metastatic squamous cell carcinoma of the head and neck. Front Oncol 2017;7:72.

9. Fakhry C, Zhang Q, Nguyen-Tan PF, et al. Human papillomavirus and overall survival after progression of oropharyngeal squamous cell carcinoma. J Clin Oncol 2014;32(30):3365–73.

10. Moskovitz JM, Moy J, Seiwert TY, et al. Immunotherapy for head and neck squamous cell carcinoma: a review of current and emerging therapeutic options. Oncologist 2017;22(6):680–93.

11. Price KA, Cohen EE. Current treatment options for metastatic head and neck cancer. Curr Treat Options Oncol 2012;13(1):35–46.

12. Omran AR. The epidemiologic transition: a theory of the epidemiology of population change. 1971. Milbank Q 2005;83(4):731–57.

13. Smith BD, Smith GL, Hurria A, et al. Future of cancer incidence in the United States: burdens upon an aging, changing nation. J Clin Oncol 2009;27(17): 2758–65.

14. Erikson C, Salsberg E, Forte G, et al. Future supply and demand for oncologists: challenges to assuring access to oncology services. J Oncol Pract 2007;3(2): 79–86.

15. VanderWalde NA, Fleming M, Weiss J, et al. Treatment of older patients with head and neck cancer: a review. Oncologist 2013;18(5):568–78.

16. Decoster L. Geriatric oncology and supportive care: a global approach to advance the science. Belg J Med Oncol 2016;10(3):108–9.

17. Pignon JP, le Maitre A, Maillard E, et al, MACH-NC Collaborative Group. Meta-analysis of chemotherapy in head and neck cancer (MACH-NC): an update on 93 randomised trials and 17,346 patients. Radiother Oncol 2009;92(1):4–14.

18. Riley GF, Lubitz JD. Long-term trends in Medicare payments in the last year of life. Health Serv Res 2010;45(2):565–76.

19. Earle CC, Neville BA, Landrum MB, et al. Trends in the aggressiveness of cancer care near the end of life. J Clin Oncol 2004;22(2):315–21.

20. Kwok AC, Semel ME, Lipsitz SR, et al. The intensity and variation of surgical care at the end of life: a retrospective cohort study. Lancet 2011;378(9800):1408–13.

21. Schenker Y, Arnold RM, Bauman JE, et al. An enhanced role for palliative care in the multidisciplinary approach to high-risk head and neck cancer. Cancer 2016; 122(3):340–3.

22. Chassin MR, Galvin RW. The urgent need to improve health care quality. Institute of Medicine National Roundtable on Health Care Quality. JAMA 1998;280(11): 1000–5.

23. Maggiore R, Zumsteg ZS, BrintzenhofeSzoc K, et al. The older adult with locoregionally advanced head and neck squamous cell carcinoma: knowledge gaps and future direction in assessment and treatment. Int J Radiat Oncol Biol Phys 2017;98(4):868–83.

24. Fried LP, Ferrucci L, Darer J, et al. Untangling the concepts of disability, frailty, and comorbidity: implications for improved targeting and care. J Gerontol A Biol Sci Med Sci 2004;59(3):255–63.

25. Rodriguez-Manas L, Feart C, Mann G, et al. Searching for an operational definition of frailty: a Delphi method based consensus statement: the frailty operative

definition-consensus conference project. J Gerontol A Biol Sci Med Sci 2013; 68(1):62–7.

26. Dent E, Kowal P, Hoogendijk EO. Frailty measurement in research and clinical practice: a review. Eur J Intern Med 2016;31:3–10.

27. Yates JW, Chalmer B, McKegney FP. Evaluation of patients with advanced cancer using the Karnofsky performance status. Cancer 1980;45(8):2220–4.

28. Oken MM, Creech RH, Tormey DC, et al. Toxicity and response criteria of the Eastern Cooperative Oncology Group. Am J Clin Oncol 1982;5(6):649–55.

29. Devons CA. Comprehensive geriatric assessment: making the most of the aging years. Curr Opin Clin Nutr Metab Care 2002;5(1):19–24.

30. Stuck AE, Siu AL, Wieland GD, et al. Comprehensive geriatric assessment: a meta-analysis of controlled trials. Lancet 1993;342(8878):1032–6.

31. Chaibi P, Magne N, Breton S, et al. Influence of geriatric consultation with comprehensive geriatric assessment on final therapeutic decision in elderly cancer patients. Crit Rev Oncol Hematol 2011;79(3):302–7.

32. Hurria A, Mohile S, Gajra A, et al. Validation of a prediction tool for chemotherapy toxicity in older adults with cancer. J Clin Oncol 2016;34(20):2366–71.

33. Bellera CA, Rainfray M, Mathoulin-Pelissier S, et al. Screening older cancer patients: first evaluation of the G-8 geriatric screening tool. Ann Oncol 2012;23(8): 2166–72.

34. Overcash JA, Beckstead J, Moody L, et al. The abbreviated comprehensive geriatric assessment (aCGA) for use in the older cancer patient as a prescreen: scoring and interpretation. Crit Rev Oncol Hematol 2006;59(3):205–10.

35. Bielderman A, van der Schans CP, van Lieshout MR, et al. Multidimensional structure of the Groningen frailty indicator in community-dwelling older people. BMC Geriatr 2013;13:86.

36. Saliba D, Elliott M, Rubenstein LZ, et al. The vulnerable elders survey: a tool for identifying vulnerable older people in the community. J Am Geriatr Soc 2001; 49(12):1691–9.

37. Neve M, Jameson MB, Govender S, et al. Impact of geriatric assessment on the management of older adults with head and neck cancer: a pilot study. J Geriatr Oncol 2016;7(6):457–62.

38. Pottel L, Lycke M, Boterberg T, et al. G-8 indicates overall and quality-adjusted survival in older head and neck cancer patients treated with curative radiochemotherapy. BMC Cancer 2015;15:875.

39. Pottel L, Lycke M, Boterberg T, et al. Serial comprehensive geriatric assessment in elderly head and neck cancer patients undergoing curative radiotherapy identifies evolution of multidimensional health problems and is indicative of quality of life. Eur J Cancer Care (Engl) 2014;23(3):401–12.

40. The National Comprehensive Cancer Network (NCCN) clinical practice guidelines in oncology. Older adult oncology. 2017. Available at: https://www.nccn.org/professionals/physician_gls/pdf/senior.pdf. Accessed October 15, 2017.

41. Walter LC, Covinsky KE. Cancer screening in elderly patients: a framework for individualized decision making. JAMA 2001;285(21):2750–6.

42. Covinsky KE, Justice AC, Rosenthal GE, et al. Measuring prognosis and case mix in hospitalized elders. The importance of functional status. J Gen Intern Med 1997;12(4):203–8.

43. Inouye SK, Peduzzi PN, Robison JT, et al. Importance of functional measures in predicting mortality among older hospitalized patients. JAMA 1998;279(15):1187–93.

44. Sessums LL, Zembrzuska H, Jackson JL. Does this patient have medical decision-making capacity? JAMA 2011;306(4):420–7.

45. Levit L, Balogh E, Nass S, et al. Delivering high-quality cancer care: charting a new course for a system in crisis. Washington, DC: National Academies Press; 2013.
46. Beswick DM, Gooding WE, Johnson JT, et al. Temporal patterns of head and neck squamous cell carcinoma recurrence with positron-emission tomography/computed tomography monitoring. Laryngoscope 2012;122(7):1512–7.
47. Ritoe SC, Krabbe PF, Kaanders JH, et al. Value of routine follow-up for patients cured of laryngeal carcinoma. Cancer 2004;101(6):1382–9.
48. Nilsen ML, Johnson JT. Potential for low-value palliative care of patients with recurrent head and neck cancer. Lancet Oncol 2017;18(5):e284–9.
49. Prigerson HG, Bao Y, Shah MA, et al. Chemotherapy use, performance status, and quality of life at the end of life. JAMA Oncol 2015;1(6):778–84.
50. O'Neill CB, Baxi SS, Atoria CL, et al. Treatment-related toxicities in older adults with head and neck cancer: a population-based analysis. Cancer 2015;121(12):2083–9.
51. Sachdev S, Refaat T, Bacchus ID, et al. Age most significant predictor of requiring enteral feeding in head-and-neck cancer patients. Radiat Oncol 2015;10:93.
52. Cruz-Jentoft AJ, Baeyens JP, Bauer JM, et al. Sarcopenia: European consensus on definition and diagnosis: report of the European Working Group on sarcopenia in older people. Age Ageing 2010;39(4):412–23.
53. Evans WJ. Skeletal muscle loss: cachexia, sarcopenia, and inactivity. Am J Clin Nutr 2010;91(4):1123S–7S.
54. Grossberg AJ, Chamchod S, Fuller CD, et al. Association of body composition with survival and locoregional control of radiotherapy-treated head and neck squamous cell carcinoma. JAMA Oncol 2016;2(6):782–9.
55. Haisfield-Wolfe ME, McGuire DB, Soeken K, et al. Prevalence and correlates of depression among patients with head and neck cancer: a systematic review of implications for research. Oncol Nurs Forum 2009;36(3):E107–25.
56. Barber B, Dergousoff J, Slater L, et al. Depression and survival in patients with head and neck cancer: a systematic review. JAMA Otolaryngol Head Neck Surg 2016;142(3):284–8.
57. Misono S, Weiss NS, Fann JR, et al. Incidence of suicide in persons with cancer. J Clin Oncol 2008;26(29):4731–8.
58. The National Comprehensive Cancer Network (NCCN) clinical practice guidelines in oncology. Palliative care. 2017. Available at: https://www.nccn.org/professionals/physician_gls/pdf/palliative.pdf. Accessed October 15, 2017.
59. Bakitas MA, Tosteson TD, Li Z, et al. Early versus delayed initiation of concurrent palliative oncology care: patient outcomes in the ENABLE III randomized controlled trial. J Clin Oncol 2015;33(13):1438–45.
60. Dionne-Odom JN, Azuero A, Lyons KD, et al. Benefits of early versus delayed palliative care to informal family caregivers of patients with advanced cancer: outcomes from the ENABLE III randomized controlled trial. J Clin Oncol 2015;33(13):1446–52.
61. Temel JS, Greer JA, Admane S, et al. Longitudinal perceptions of prognosis and goals of therapy in patients with metastatic non-small-cell lung cancer: results of a randomized study of early palliative care. J Clin Oncol 2011;29(17):2319–26.
62. The SHARE approach. Available at: https://www.ahrq.gov/professionals/education/curriculum-tools/shareddecisionmaking/index.html. Accessed October 15, 2017.
63. Stacey D, Legare F, Col NF, et al. Decision aids for people facing health treatment or screening decisions. Cochrane Database Syst Rev 2014;(1):CD001431.

64. Levinson W, Kao A, Kuby A, et al. Not all patients want to participate in decision making. A national study of public preferences. J Gen Intern Med 2005;20(6): 531–5.

65. Chawla N, Arora NK. Why do some patients prefer to leave decisions up to the doctor: lack of self-efficacy or a matter of trust? J Cancer Surviv 2013;7(4): 592–601.

66. Becerra Perez MM, Menear M, Brehaut JC, et al. Extent and predictors of decision regret about health care decisions: a systematic review. Med Decis Making 2016;36(6):777–90.

67. Goepfert RP, Fuller CD, Gunn GB, et al. Symptom burden as a driver of decisional regret in long-term oropharyngeal carcinoma survivors. Head Neck 2017;39(11): 2151–8.

68. Broeckaert B, Glare P. Ethical perspectives. In: Glare P, Christakis NA, editors. Prognosis in advanced cancer. New York: Oxford University Press Inc; 2008. p. 89–94.

69. Christakis NA, Lamont EB. Extent and determinants of error in doctors' prognoses in terminally ill patients: prospective cohort study. BMJ 2000;320(7233):469–72.

70. Jalukar V, Funk GF, Christensen AJ, et al. Health states following head and neck cancer treatment: patient, health-care professional, and public perspectives. Head Neck 1998;20(7):600–8.

71. Mohide EA, Archibald SD, Tew M, et al. Postlaryngectomy quality-of-life dimensions identified by patients and health care professionals. Am J Surg 1992; 164(6):619–22.

72. Otto RA, Dobie RA, Lawrence V, et al. Impact of a laryngectomy on quality of life: perspective of the patient versus that of the health care provider. Ann Otol Rhinol Laryngol 1997;106(8):693–9.

73. Kruser JM, Nabozny MJ, Steffens NM, et al. "Best case/worst case": qualitative evaluation of a novel communication tool for difficult in-the-moment surgical decisions. J Am Geriatr Soc 2015;63(9):1805–11.

74. Hall DE, Arya S, Schmid KK, et al. Development and initial validation of the risk analysis index for measuring frailty in surgical populations. JAMA Surg 2017; 152(2):175–82.

Cutaneous Head and Neck Malignancies in the Elderly

Brian B. Hughley, MD[a],*, Cecelia E. Schmalbach, MD, MS[b]

KEYWORDS

- Cutaneous • Malignancy • Geriatric • Elderly • Skin cancer
- Multidisciplinary treatment

KEY POINTS

- Management of cutaneous head and neck malignancy in the elderly requires a multidisciplinary approach tailored to each individual.
- The incidence of cutaneous malignancies in the elderly is increasing.
- In most cases, first-line treatment of cutaneous malignancies is surgical.
- Radiotherapy and/or chemotherapy are often used as adjuvant therapy but in selected cases may be used as first-line therapy.

Cutaneous head and neck malignancies are primarily diseases of the geriatric population. Although adjuvant treatments, such as radiation, chemotherapy, monoclonal antibodies, and immunotherapy, have a role, the primary treatment of all types remains surgical. Elderly patients are more likely to have comorbidities that increase their perioperative risks. Several preoperative risk assessment tools have been developed to help stratify general postoperative risk based on frailty. However, none of these are specific to head and neck surgery.

Most head and neck cutaneous malignancies are relatively small and involve skin-only excision with minor local reconstruction. However, at times, more invasive surgery is required, such as neck dissection, parotidectomy, lateral temporal bone resection, or major free tissue transfer reconstruction. Although advanced age itself is not a contraindication for any of these procedures, the perioperative risks associated with many of the comorbidities present in the geriatric population have led to the investigation of other treatment modalities. Radiation therapy, chemotherapy,

The authors have no financial conflicts of interest. No funding was provided for this work.
[a] Otolaryngology–Head and Neck Surgery, University of Alabama at Birmingham, BDB 563, 1720 2nd Avenue South, Birmingham, AL 35294-0012, USA; [b] Otolaryngology–Head and Neck Surgery, Head and Neck–Microvascular Surgery, Clinical Affairs, Indiana University School of Medicine, Fesler Hall, 1130 W. Michigan Street, Suite 400, Indianapolis, IN 46202, USA
* Corresponding author.
E-mail address: bhughley@uabmc.edu

Clin Geriatr Med 34 (2018) 245–258
https://doi.org/10.1016/j.cger.2018.01.004
0749-0690/18/© 2018 Elsevier Inc. All rights reserved.

monoclonal antibodies, and immunologic treatments are all used to varying degrees in cutaneous malignancies; although they all have associated risks, they may be tolerated in selected geriatric patients.

The 4 most common types of cutaneous head and neck malignancies are presented in the following sections, with background information, demographics, and treatment options discussed. Special considerations of the geriatric population are discussed for each.

NONMELANOMA SKIN CANCER

Basal cell carcinoma (BCC) and cutaneous squamous cell carcinoma (cSCC) are the two most common malignancies in the United States.[1,2] They are frequently referred to together as nonmelanoma skin cancer (NMSC). Although NMSCs are not included in most major cancer registries, in 2012 there were an estimated 2.8 million new diagnoses of BCC and 700,000 of cSCC.[3] In fact, the incidence of cSCC has increased 200% over the past 30 years. Despite the overall favorable prognosis of most NMSCs, 10% will recur and 3% to 5% are associated with regional or distant metastasis.[4,5] As the risk of NMSC is associated with cumulative sun exposure, the light-skinned geriatric population is at significantly higher risk. It is estimated that 40% to 50% of Americans will have at least one NMSC by 65 years of age.[6] This finding creates a significant economic health care impact, with $4.8 billion per year spent treating NMSC in the United States.[7] Although many similarities exist in the treatment options for BCC and cSCC, there are several differences, especially regarding nonsurgical therapy. NMSC are diseases primarily of the geriatric population, and multidisciplinary care and management plays an important role.

Basal Cell Carcinoma

BCC is the most common cancer in the United States; it is in fact more common than all other cancers combined and twice as common as cSCC, which is the second most common cancer.[8] BCC risk is related to cumulative sun exposure and is, therefore, high in the geriatric light-skinned population.[9] BCC is more common in men, and the incidence in the geriatric population is increasing. Regional and distant metastasis from BCC is very rare and reported to occur in less than 0.1% of cases.[10] The relative 5-year survival is 99%. Despite this favorable prognosis, if left untreated, BCCs of the head and neck can be locally destructive; surgical treatment can be associated with significant functional and cosmetic difficulties.

Risks factors for aggressive BCCs include diameter greater than 2 cm, location in the H region of the face, incomplete prior excision, long-standing presence, perineural invasion, and aggressive histologic subtype (morpheaform and basosquamous)[9] (**Table 1**). Other risk factors for BCC include UV exposure, radiation exposure, immunosuppression, and human immunodeficiency virus (HIV)+ status.[11] Although still unlikely to be associated with distant spread, these lesions may be locally invasive and may end up extending farther than is evident clinically, resulting in larger surgical defects. In general, treatment of small, superficial BCC is tolerated well in elderly patients; however, larger more aggressive lesions may require multi-modality treatment, which can be challenging in the geriatric population.

Histologic subtypes of BCC associated with aggressive tumor behavior include the morpheaform, basosquamous, sclerosing, and mixed infiltrative types.[12] Excision is the recommended treatment of BCC.[13] For low-risk lesions, curettage or electrodessication may be considered. Photodynamic therapy may also be an option for thin superficial and nodular BCCs.[14] This procedure is generally tolerated well, and treatment

Table 1
Nonmelanoma skin cancer high-risk features

	Low Risk	High Risk
Location/size	<20 mm Area L <10 mm Area M <6 mm Area H	≥20 mm Area L ≥10 mm Area M ≥6 mm Area H
Boarders	Well defined	Poorly defined
History	Primary tumor	Recurrent tumor
Immunosuppression	No	Yes
Prior radiation	No	Yes
Pathology	BCC: nodular; superficial	BCC: morpheaform; basosquamous, sclerosing; micronodular SCC: acantholytic; adenosquamous; desmoplastic; metaplastic

Abbreviations: Area H, mask area of face (central face, eyelids, eyebrows, periorbital, nose, lips, chin, mandible, preauricular/postauricular skin, ear, genitalia, hands, feet); Area L, trunk and extremities (excluding pretibial, hands, feet, nail units, and ankles); Area M, cheeks, forehead, scalp, neck, and pretibial.

Data from National Comprehensive Cancer Network clinical guidelines: Basal Cell Skin Cancer version 1.2018; and Squamous Cell Skin Cancer version 2.2018.

is performed in an outpatient setting that requires no anesthesia or sedation. Occasionally, re-excision or minor reconstruction of skin defects is required and can be performed using local anesthesia.

For high-risk BCC, complete excision with circumferential peripheral and deep margin assessment is recommended as the first-line treatment.[13] Surgery may be performed as a standard surgical excision with 4-mm or larger margins or by the Mohs technique. Reconstruction of the defect is often required. If standard surgical excision is performed, complex tissue rearrangement should not be performed until complete histologic analysis of all margins is complete. Simple skin graft or primary closure may be performed, as long as the orientation and correlation with any potential positive margins are possible. Delayed reconstruction is often required because of margin analysis or patient/surgeon scheduling and is not associated with any wound complications.[15]

Mohs surgery and most standard surgical excisions of BCCs are performed with local anesthesia or light sedation. This sedation is well tolerated by most patients, including elderly patients, and is safe for those with multiple medical comorbidities. Occasionally, larger resections or more complex reconstructions require general anesthesia that may not be safe for certain patients. In patients unable to undergo surgical excision, radiation therapy may be considered. Recent data show that radiation therapy is safe and effective for head and neck BCCs as definitive treatment or adjuvant treatment of highly aggressive lesions.[16] Primary radiation may be effective for patients in whom surgery is contraindicated or if the functional/cosmetic outcomes following excision are unacceptable.

Although rare, BCC can occasionally present as a large, destructive lesion requiring free tissue transfer for reconstruction following resection. These surgical procedures require a long general anesthetic and an intense postoperative course. Recent evaluation of a relatively large cohort of these patients (mean age of 64 years) showed very low morbidity, with no serious complications.[17] Aggressive lesions with bone (mandible and calvarium) involvement had similar overall survival and disease-free survival (DFS). Adjuvant radiation increased DFS by more than 1 year. The investigators concluded that resection and reconstruction of aggressive BCC, even in the geriatric patient population, should still be considered first-line therapy.

Occasionally patients will have recalcitrant BCC, which fails surgical and/or radiation therapy. Systemic agents have recently been approved for the treatment of unresectable, locally advanced or metastatic BCC. Vismodegib (Erividge) is a hedgehog signaling pathway targeted agent approved in 2012 for BCC. It is indicated for adjuvant therapy in the setting of unresectable disease and the rare case of metastatic BCC.[13] In these cases, consultation with a multidisciplinary tumor board is recommended as well as consideration of a clinical trial when possible.

Overall, vismodegib is reasonably well tolerated, even in the geriatric population. Side effects include arthralgias, muscle cramping, alopecia, fatigue, and loss of appetite with weight loss.[18] Although side effects are typically minor, 30% to 40% of patients will require a drug holiday. Vismodegib has successfully been used in the geriatric patient population. The development of the hedgehog signaling pathway inhibitors is a major advance in the treatment of nonresectable, locally advanced, and metastatic BCC. Long-term data regarding the durability of treatment, adverse effects, and use as an adjuvant/neoadjuvant agent remain to be elucidated.[19]

Squamous Cell Carcinoma

cSCC is the second most common malignancy in the United States. Although many of the high-risk features are similar to BCC, cSCC is much more likely to be regionally or distantly metastatic (see **Table 1**). For this reason, treatment recommendations often involve more aggressive procedures, including parotidectomy and/or neck dissection. Although these procedures are generally well tolerated, geriatric patients are at higher risk for perioperative mortality and complications.[20] All of the treatment modalities should be considered, ideally in a multidisciplinary tumor board setting, in order to determine the extent and combinations of surgery, radiation, and systemic therapy appropriate for each advanced case.

Chronic sunlight exposure is the main risk factor for cSCC. Therefore, older patients, especially those who have worked in outdoor occupations, carry a higher risk. Chronic immunosuppression is also associated with an increased risk of cSCC, including solid organ transplantation, lymphoma, and HIV.[21–23] Other risk factors for aggressive, recurrent, or metastatic disease include location in a site of a chronic wound or prior radiation therapy, greater than a 2-mm depth of invasion, poorly differentiated histology, and perineural invasion.[24]

Radiologic imaging of the primary site and regional lymph nodes is appropriate in aggressive cSCC. If there is concern for underlying bone invasion or if the deep extent of the primary tumor cannot be determined, CT of the primary and neck is appropriate.[25] If neurologic symptoms are present or if there is concern for dura invasion, MRI should be obtained.[26] Patients with a greater than 2-cm primary tumor size are at high risk for metastasis and warrant imaging of the parotid and cervical nodal basins for regional staging.[27]

For low-risk, localized cSCC, local excision is the standard of care.[27] Local excision may be accomplished by curettage and electrodessication provided the lesion does not extend into the subcutaneous tissue and is not located in hair-bearing skin. The procedure is performed with local anesthesia and is well tolerated by geriatric patients who are unable to undergo general anesthesia presuming cosmetic and functional considerations are minimal. Full surgical excision with 4- to 6-mm clinical margins is an alternative option for these low-risk lesions and may be performed as standard surgical excision or the Mohs technique.[27] Full circumferential peripheral and deep margin assessment is recommended. Patients older than 60 years who are unable or unwilling to undergo surgical excision may receive localized radiation treatment to the primary cSCC site.

Excision with complete circumferential and peripheral margin assessment is recommended for high-risk cSCC.[27] Again, this procedure may be accomplished with either standard surgical or the Mohs technique. If standard surgical excision is performed, full margin assessment should be complete before any complex reconstruction, which could make identification and reresection of positive margins challenging. Surgical defects may require complex skin rearrangement, pedicled flaps, or free tissue transfer (**Fig. 1**). Patients may require a long general anesthetic or multiple episodes of general anesthesia. Such considerations should be factored into the decision to perform surgery and the potential for multiple surgeries discussed beforehand.

Radiation therapy may also be considered as a primary treatment of high-risk cSCC, especially if patients are medically unable or unwilling to undergo surgical excision with associated reconstruction.[28] The side effects of radiation therapy are not insignificant and, depending on location of the primary tumor, include loss of vision, dysphagia (leading to dehydration and malnutrition), skin ulceration, and pain. Additionally, radiation treatments occur most weekdays for multiple weeks, and transportation/logistics can be difficult for many infirm geriatric patients. Radiation is an effective treatment of primary, high-risk cSCC and avoids surgery with general anesthesia; however, it is also associated with many side effects that can be poorly tolerated in the same patients for whom surgery is not ideal. In these patients, multidisciplinary care is essential and should include collaboration between surgeons, radiation oncologists, social workers, and patients along with their families and caregivers.

All patients with palpable lymphadenopathy warrant further workup to include fine-needle aspiration (FNA) and dedicated imaging. Lymphadenectomy remains the standard of care for patients with metastatic, regional disease.[27] In addition, a parotidectomy is indicated if the primary tumor invades the parotid fascia or if a positive lymph node is located in the parotid gland.[24,29] A parotidectomy should also be included in the surgical plan if the primary cSCC arises superior to the parotid bed in the setting of cervical lymph node metastasis because the cSCC presumably drained through the parotid nodal basin.[24]

High-risk patients, such as the immunosuppressed with cSCC clinically and radiographically limited to the local site, may benefit from elective lymphadenectomy to include parotidectomy. These elective procedures identify occult, micrometastatic regional disease, which provides important prognostic and staging information to guide the possible need for adjuvant therapy. However, the risks of surgery and anesthesia

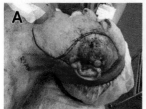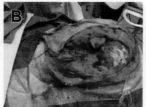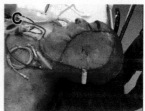

Fig. 1. An 82-year-old male solid organ transplant patient with a large, aggressive left preauricular cSCC with invasion of the parotid gland, facial nerve, and temporal bone. (*A*) Tumor before resection; (*B*) operative wound following wide local excision of skin, radical parotidectomy, left neck dissection, and left lateral temporal bone resection; (*C*) immediately following reconstruction with an anterolateral thigh free flap.

must be taken into account for the geriatric patient population. Elective parotidectomy should be considered in cSCC of the temporal region if the tumor is greater than 2 cm or if perineural or lympho-vascular invasion is noted.[30] If patients are not good candidates for elective parotidectomy, prophylactic radiation is an alternative option in these high-risk patients.[24] A recent systematic review of the literature demonstrated that sentinel node biopsy is feasible for high-risk patients with head and neck cSCC and carries a similar false rate of omission as melanoma whereby the procedure is the standard of care.[31] This staging modality may be an ideal alternative in high-risk geriatric patients because it is a shorter general anesthetic and carries a lower risk.

Adjuvant radiation therapy is recommended for patients in the setting of cSCC that is metastatic to the parotid gland, the presence of a lymph node that is greater than 3 cm, or if multiple nodes are involved.[27,32] Postoperative radiation therapy is also indicated if perineural invasion of multiple small nerves or a single large nerve is noted on histology.[33] These patients are at significant risk of local recurrence. Additionally, in the case of perineural invasion, the ipsilateral parotid and cervical nodal beds should be treated with radiation. Patients who have positive margins on final histologic analysis who are unable to undergo reresection also meet the criteria for adjuvant radiation to the primary tumor site.[24]

The role of systemic therapy in the treatment of cSCC is limited and not well defined. Distant metastasis is rare; the use of chemotherapy has been studied in large, aggressive, invasive tumors. Cisplatin can be used in combination with radiation therapy for adjuvant treatment of large, invasive tumors with positive unresectable margins or in the case of extranodal extension of cervical metastasis.[24,27] However, much of the data on this is extrapolated from the treatment of mucosal upper aerodigestive tract SCC.[34] Concurrent chemoradiation is associated with increased side effects, including myelosuppression, chronic wounds, dysphagia, gastrointestinal distress, and dehydration. However, in geriatric patients with good performance status, the treatment is well tolerated, without an increase in adverse effects compared with radiation alone.[35]

The epidermal growth factor receptor (EGFR) target cetuximab has been shown to be effective as the primary treatment of advanced, unresectable cSCC with reasonable toxicity tolerance in the elderly.[36] Gefitinib is an EGFR tyrosine kinase inhibitor that has shown efficacy in the treatment of aggressive, nonresectable, or recurrent cSCC.[37] Both cetuximab and gefitinib are associated with cutaneous and gastrointestinal toxicities but are generally tolerated better in elderly patients than platinum-based chemotherapy.

Nivolumab and pembrolizumab are both anti–programmed death-1 (PD-1) monoclonal antibodies that have shown promise in treating unresectable cSCC. These agents carry a better progression-free survival and toxicity profile when compared with platinum-based chemotherapy.[38] They are currently undergoing evaluation for the specific treatment of cSCC, and use is limited to patients who have failed standard chemotherapy agents. Ultimately, the use of any systemic agent in the treatment of advanced cSCC must be undertaken carefully and with the guidance of a multidisciplinary tumor board to include the potential for clinical trial involvement.

MERKEL CELL CARCINOMA

Merkel cell carcinoma (MCC) is an aggressive cutaneous malignancy of neuroendocrine origin common among the geriatric population.[39–41] Most patients are Caucasian. More than 50% of all MCCs occur in the head and neck, making it the most common primary tumor site.[42] MCC is associated with the polyomovirus.[43] As with NMSC, patients who are immunocompromised because of solid-organ transplant,

HIV+ status, chronic lymphocytic leukemia, multiple myeloma, and non-Hodgkin lymphoma are at a significantly higher risk.[40,44]

MCC typically presents as a painless, smooth, pink or red, firm nodule and is frequently associated with a rapid increase in size.[45] Although rare, a high index of suspicion for MCC is important when evaluating a new lesion in the head and neck of geriatric Caucasian patients; this suspicion should be even higher in immunocompromised patients. Biopsy is required for tissue diagnosis. This biopsy may be done via excisional, incisional, or punch biopsy.[46] Complete excision with wide margins is not recommended initially, as this may interfere with accurate lymphoscintigraphy and sentinel lymph node biopsy (SLNB).[47] Once a diagnosis of MCC is obtained, treatment of the primary site and regional lymph node staging (for clinically node-negative cervical and parotid lymphatics) are undertaken.

Histologic variants of MCC include trabecular, intermediate, and small cell; intermediate and small cell variants are more aggressive.[48] MCC is one of the many small blue cell neoplasms and may be difficult to accurately diagnose on hematoxylin and eosin (H&E) staining alone. Therefore, specific immunohistochemical markers are recommended: cytokeratin-20 (CK-20), synaptophysin, and chromogranin are positive in MCC, whereas thyroid transcription factor-1 (TTF-1) is negative.[49] The addition of these tests to standard H&E staining is important in verifying the diagnosis of MCC, as the treatment often differs from NMSC as well as other small blue cell neoplasms.

Complete workup of a newly diagnosed MCC includes imaging of the primary site and the lymphatic nodal basins. CT with contrast or MRI is typically used. PET/CT may be useful in cases of unknown primary MCC or recurrent MCC if regional or distant metastasis is suspected.[50] Clinically positive nodes should be biopsied with FNA.

Primary treatment of MCC is surgical excision with 1- to 2-cm margins.[47] Margins this wide may not be possible because of functional considerations, specifically near the eyelids, nares, or oral commissure. In such cases, the Mohs technique may be considered.[47,49] Primary radiation therapy may be considered in patients who are not surgical candidates or those who refuse surgery.[49] Confirmed regional metastatic MCC necessitates lymphadenectomy as described earlier in the cSCC section. Adjuvant radiation to the primary site as well as the neck/parotid is recommended.[47,49] In patients who are unable, or unwilling, to undergo surgery, primary radiation therapy may be considered, although this is likely palliative in nature.[47]

In patients with clinically node-negative lymph node basins, SLNB is considered the standard of care for regional staging.[47] Accurate regional staging is important in prognosis, as those with lymph node metastasis have a 5-year survival that can be as low as 48%.[46] Micrometastasis is difficult to detect clinically, and elective lymphadenectomy is not recommended.[47] SLNB provides the pathologist with the highest-risk lymph nodes of the first draining nodal basin. In doing so, thorough evaluation to include microsectioning and MCC-specific immunohistochemical staining (CK-20; TTF-1) can be performed to identify occult disease.[46] SLNB should be performed at the time of definitive wide local excision of the primary site in order to maintain accurate nodal drainage pathways for lymphoscintigraphy. Patients with a positive sentinel node should undergo a therapeutic neck dissection with postoperative radiation therapy.[47] Those with a negative SLNB do not require either neck dissection or radiation to the neck. SLNB remains the most sensitive modality for regional staging and allows for identification of patients who may benefit from completion lymphadenectomy with adjuvant radiation therapy. Conversely, it allows identification of those who do not need to undergo neck dissection, thus, avoiding a major, potentially unnecessary, head and neck operation in this predominantly elderly population.

Systemic therapy has a limited role in the treatment of MCC. Studies have not shown an increase in overall survival with the addition of chemotherapy to adjuvant radiation therapy. However, combination chemotherapy of cisplatin or carboplatin plus etoposide is occasionally used along with radiation in cases of widespread disease. These agents may be used alone in nonsurgical patients for palliation. Topotecan may also be used in the geriatric population.[51] The toxicity of adding chemotherapy to radiation therapy in older patients is significant and may preclude its use. The use of chemotherapy in the treatment of MCC should carefully be considered on an individual patient basis, ideally in the setting of a multidisciplinary tumor board.

CUTANEOUS MELANOMA

The incidence of cutaneous melanoma continues to increase at epidemic proportions, with an estimated 87,110 new cases in the United States in 2017.[52] The associated mortality rate continues to increase at approximately 3% per year, and melanoma remains the most lethal form of cutaneous cancer. Whereas BCC and cSCC are associated with cumulative exposure to UV radiation, melanoma is associated with intense, intermittent sun exposure causing blistering sunburns.

The American Cancer Society has coined the educational ABCDE acronym, which highlights the following concerning features: lesion Asymmetry, Border irregularity, Color variation within a lesion, Diameter greater than 6 mm, and Evolution/change of a lesion.[53,54] It is important to note that a subset of melanomas, including the nodular, amelanotic, and desmoplastic melanomas, lack these common features of the ABCDs. Any pigmented lesion meeting the aforementioned criteria warrants biopsy.

Cutaneous melanoma remains a surgical disease. Wide local excision of the primary melanoma is warranted, with surgical margins based on primary tumor depth of invasion (Table 2). Therefore, Mohs microsurgery is not considered the standard of care for melanoma. Intraoperative frozen section analysis of margins is also discouraged because of the high false-positive rates.[55] Because of this, a second staged, delayed reconstruction is recommended after the final pathologic analysis of the margins, unless simple reconstruction, such as primary closure or skin grafting, is feasible.[56] Any immediate reconstruction should allow for reliable identification of all portions of the original margins, so that reresection is accurate and as limited as is oncologically sound.

Defects following melanoma resection are often treated with local tissue rearrangement for cosmetic and functional purposes. Delayed reconstruction necessitates multiple anesthetics. This requirement can be a consideration in geriatric patients who

Table 2 National Comprehensive Cancer Network recommendations for surgical margins in cutaneous melanoma	
Tumor Thickness	Clinical Margin Recommendation
In situ	0.5–1.0 cm
≤1.0 mm	1.0 cm
1.01–2.0 mm	1.0–2.0 cm
2.01–4.0 mm	2.0 cm
>4.0 mm	2.0 cm

Data from National Comprehensive Cancer Network clinical practice guidelines in oncology: melanoma; version I.2017. 2016.

may require longer recovery from even a short general anesthetic. Fortunately, many scalp and facial resections, as well as reconstructive procedures, can be performed under local anesthesia only or monitored anesthesia with intravenous sedation. In patients with severe cardiac or pulmonary disease, consideration may be given to simpler, single-stage reconstruction at the expense of cosmesis if a single procedure with simple reconstruction (eg, skin graft) would be safer.

Elective neck dissection/lymphadenectomy is no longer considered the standard of care in patients with high-risk localized disease, and it has been replaced by SLNB.[56–58] The current guidelines from the National Comprehensive Cancer Network recommend SLNB for melanomas based on the depth of invasion and high-risk features (**Table 3**). For thin melanomas (depth of invasion 0.75 mm–0.99 mm), SLNB should be considered if poor prognostic features are present, including mitotic rate greater than 1 mm^2, ulceration, young age, and regression. In the geriatric population, however, SLNB may be considered when pathologic high-risk features are present in thin primary tumors. SLNB is recommended for patients with localized, intermediate-thickness melanomas (1–4 mm) as well as for thick melanomas (>4 mm).[59] These important prognostic features highlight the need for patients with a suspected melanoma to undergo a 2-staged process to include (1) a punch biopsy or narrow margin excisional biopsy as opposed to shave biopsy or wide local excision and (2) definitive treatment with wide local excision and associated SLNB if indicated.

Patients with a negative SLNB are followed closely for recurrence. Traditionally, patients with a positive SLNB are returned to the operating room within 2 weeks for completion lymphadenectomy and parotidectomy if warranted. Recent results of the international Multicenter Selective Lymphadenectomy Trial II question the utility for this additional surgery.[60] In an attempt to determine if SLNB is both diagnostic as well as therapeutic, patients with one positive sentinel lymph node were randomized to observation with serial ultrasound versus completion lymphadenectomy. The 3-year melanoma-specific survival was similar between the surgery and observations arms (68% vs 86%; $P = .42$). However, the surgery arm experienced an improved DFS (68% vs 64%; $P = .05$) and regional control (92% vs 77%; $P<.001$). This improved DFS was at the expense of lymphedema, which was significantly higher in the surgery arm compared with the observation arm (24.1% vs 6.3%; $P<.001$). However, lymphedema is a known complication of groin and extremity complete lymph node dissection but does not carry the same risk in the head and neck region.

Table 3	
National Comprehensive Cancer Network recommendations for sentinel lymph node biopsy in cutaneous melanoma	
Tumor Depth of Invasion	**SLNB Recommendation**
<0.75 mm without high-risk features[a]	Not recommended
<0.75 mm with high-risk features	May be considered
0.75–1.00 mm without high-risk features	May be considered
0.75–1.00 mm with high-risk features	Recommended
>1.00 mm	Recommended
Pure desmoplastic melanoma	May be considered
Mixed desmoplastic melanoma	Recommended

[a] High-risk features include Clark level, mitotic rate, ulceration, lympho-vascular invasion, young age, and regression.

Data from National Comprehensive Cancer Network clinical practice guidelines in oncology: melanoma; version I.2017. 2016.

All patients presenting with melanoma and palpable lymphadenopathy warrant FNA of the mass and dedicated radiographic imaging. It is important to remember that melanoma has a propensity for brain metastasis, and MRI is recommended in the setting of advanced disease.[57] Similar to both cSCC and MCC, lymphadenectomy with or without parotidectomy remains the standard of care in the treatment of regional metastasis.[57]

Adjuvant radiotherapy has a limited role in the treatment of melanoma. Postoperative radiation to the primary site can be considered in desmoplastic melanoma, which has a propensity for neural spread as well as recurrent disease. Regional metastasis to the parotid or cervical nodes may also be treated with adjuvant radiotherapy. The criteria include 1 or more parotid node regardless of size, 2 or more cervical nodes or 1 cervical node 3 cm or greater in size, 2 or more axillary nodes or any axillary node 4 cm or greater in size, and 3 or more inguinal nodes or any inguinal node 4 cm or greater in size. The acute and late toxicities should be strongly considered, especially in the elderly. Regional control has been shown to be improved with adjuvant neck radiation, but no survival benefit has been shown. In geriatric patients, this should be considered on an individual basis, through discussion at a multidisciplinary tumor board. Radiation may also be considered in cases of unresectable disease with the intent of palliative treatment.[57]

Despite surgical resection, patients with localized stage II or regional stage III melanoma continue to have a significant risk of recurrence, both locally and systemically. Traditionally high-dose interferon alpha 2b has been used in this context for the past 2 decades. The treatment carries significant side effects, including fatigue, fevers, debilitating myalgias, and even suicidal ideation, all of which must be taken into account for geriatric patients. A 2013 Cochrane systematic review confirmed the benefit of adjuvant interferon alpha 2b but failed to identify either subsets of patients or treatment variants that benefited preferentially.[61] Currently, interferon should be considered for patients with thicker T3 ulcerated lesions, T4 lesions, regional metastasis, in-transit metastasis, or recurrent disease.[57,61]

Many recent advancements have been made in systemic therapy for metastatic and unresectable melanoma. Through various mechanisms, these drugs work to enhance the body's immune response. Decline in function of the immune system with age is potentially related to worse outcomes in elderly patients with melanoma.[62] Unfortunately, drugs that boost the immune response to tumor cells are also associated with toxicities not well tolerated in the geriatric population, such as immune-mediated dermatitis, decreased appetite, arthralgia, cough, and diarrhea.

Systemic agents used for advanced melanoma include pembrolizumab and nivolumab, which are monoclonal antibodies that target the protein PD-1 on T cells. Ipilimumab blocks CTLA-4, another T-cell component, to also boost the immune response. Nivolumab/ipilimumab combination therapy has been shown to increase the overall response rate and progression-free survival in patients with metastatic melanoma, but this is associated with higher toxicity rates than either drug alone.[63]

Dabrafenib and vemurafenib are oral agents that target BRAF gene mutations that are present in 50% of melanomas. These agents can be combined with trametinib or cobemetinib, which block MEK proteins, a downstream pathway product of the BRAF mutation. Dabrafenib/trametinib and vemurafenib/cobemetinib combination therapy has shown increased DFS and overall survival in patients with BRAF-positive unresectable stage IV disease.[64] The increased toxicity of combination therapy, especially in patients with cardiac, respiratory, or renal disease, should be considered in geriatric patients from a multidisciplinary standpoint.

SUMMARY

Cutaneous cancers are a common entity within the geriatric population, especially because of the association of cumulative exposure to UV radiation from the sun. The most common entities are BCC, cSCC, melanoma, and MCC. As the incidence of cutaneous cancers continues to increase, it is important to educate patients and physicians on the importance of sun avoidance, appropriate needs for biopsy, and evidence-based algorithms for staging and subsequent treatment. Given the complex comorbidities unique to the geriatric population, multidisciplinary care, ideally in the setting of a dedicated oncology board, is imperative.

REFERENCES

1. Miller DL, Weinstock MA. Nonmelanoma skin cancer in the United States: incidence. J AM Acad Dermatol 1994;30:774778.
2. Asgari MM, Moffet HH, Ray GT, et al. Trends in basal cell carcinoma incidence and identification of high-risk subgroups, 1998-2012. JAMA Dermatol 2015; 151:976–81.
3. Karia PS, Han J, Schmults CD. Cutaneous squamous cell carcinoma: estimated incidence of disease, nodal metastasis, and deaths from disease in the United States, 2012. J Am Acad Dermatol 2013;68:957–66.
4. von Domarus H, Stevens PJ. Metastatic basal cell carcinoma: report of five cases and review of 170 cases in the literature. J Am Acad Dermatol 1984; 10:1043–60.
5. Nguyen-Nielsen M, Wang L, Pedersen L, et al. The incidence of metastatic basal cell carcinoma in Denmark, 1997-2010. Eur J Dermatol 2015;25:463–8.
6. NCI cancer trends 2009/2010. Available at: https://progressreport.cancer.gov/sites/default/files/archive/report2009.pdf. Accessed November 9, 2017.
7. Guy GP, Berkowitz Z, Jones SE, et al. State indoor tanning laws and adolescent indoor tanning. Am J Public Health 2014;104(4):69–74.
8. Siegel RL, Miller KD, Jemal A. Cancer statistics, 2016. CA Cancer J Clin 2016;66: 7–30.
9. Roewert-Huber J, Lange-Asschenfeldt B, Stockfleth E, et al. Epidemiology and aetiology of basal cell carcinoma. Br J Dermatol 2007;157:47–51.
10. Weissferdt A, Kalhor N, Moran CA. Cutaneous basal cell carcinoma with distant metastasis to thorax and bone. Virchows Arch 2017;470:687–94.
11. de Sa TRC, Silva R, Lopes JM. Basal cell carcinoma of the skin (part 1): epidemiology, pathology, and genetic syndromes. Future Oncol 2015;11:3011–21.
12. Bartos V, Pokorny D, Zacharova O, et al. Recurrent basal cell carcinoma: a clinicopathological study and evaluation of histomorphological findings in primary and recurrent lesions. Acta Dermatovenerol Alp Pannonica Adriat 2011;20:67–75.
13. National Comprehensive Cancer Network Clinical practice guidelines in oncology: basal cell skin cancer; version 1.2018. 2017.
14. Jerjes W, Hamdoon Z, Hopper C. Photodynamic therapy in the management of basal cell carcinoma: retrospective evaluation of outcome. Photodiagnosis Photodyn Ther 2017;19:22–7.
15. Miller MQ, David AP, McLean JE, et al. Association of Mohs reconstructive surgery timing with postoperative complications. JAMA Facial Plast Surg 2017 [Epub ahead of print]. Available at: https://jamanetwork.com/journals/jamafacialplasticsurgery/article-abstract/2653281?redirect=true. Accessed October 28, 2017.

16. Rishi A, Huang SH, O'Sullivan B, et al. Outcome following radiotherapy for head and neck basal cell carcinoma with 'aggressive' features. Oral Oncol 2017;72: 157–64.

17. Burch MB, Chung TK, Rosenthal EL, et al. Multimodality management of high-risk head and neck basal cell carcinoma requiring free-flap reconstruction. Otolaryngol Head Neck Surg 2015;152(5):868–73.

18. Sekulic A, Migden MR, Oro AE, et al. Efficacy and safety of vismodegib in advanced basal-cell carcinoma. N Engl J Med 2012;366:2171–9.

19. Apalla Z, Papageorgiou C, Lallas A. Spotlight on vismodegib in the treatment of basal cell carcinoma: an evidence-based review of its place in therapy. Clin Cosmet Investig Dermatol 2017;10:171–7.

20. Deiner S, Westlake B, Dutton RP. Patterns of surgical care and complications in the elderly. J Am Geriatr Soc 2014;62:829–45.

21. Jensen AO, Svaerke C, Farkas D, et al. Skin cancer risk among solid organ recipients: a nationwide cohort study in Denmark. Acta Derm Venereol 2010;90:474–9.

22. Brewer JD, Shanafelt TD, Khezri F, et al. Increased incidence and recurrence rates of nonmelanoma skin cancer in patients with non-Hodgkin lymphoma: a Rochester, MN epidemiology project population-based study. J Am Acad Dermatol 2015;72:302–9.

23. Silverberg MJ, Leyden W, Warton EM, et al. HIV infection status, immunodeficiency, and the incidence of non-melanoma skin cancer. J Natl Cancer Inst 2013;105:350–60.

24. Ow TJ, Wang HR, McLellan B, et al. AHNS series—do you know your guidelines: diagnosis and management of cutaneous squamous cell carcinoma. Head Neck 2016;38(11):1589–95.

25. Humphreys TR, Shah K, Wysong A, et al. The role of imaging in the management of patients with nonmelanoma skin cancer: when is imaging necessary? J Am Acad Dermatol 2017;76(4):591–607.

26. Williams LS, Mancuso AA, Mendenhall WM. Perineural spread of cutaneous squamous and basal cell carcinoma: CT and MR detection and its impact on patient management and prognosis. Int J Radiat Oncol Biol Phys 2001;49(4): 1061–9.

27. National Comprehensive Cancer Network clinical practice guidelines in oncology: Squamous cell skin cancer; version 2.2018. 2017.

28. Cognetta AB, Howard BM, Heaton HP, et al. Superficial x-ray in the treatment of basal and squamous cell carcinomas: a viable option in select patients. J Am Acad Dermatol 2012;67:1235–41.

29. Sweeny L, Zimmerman T, Carroll WR, et al. Head and neck cutaneous squamous cell carcinoma requiring parotidectomy: prognostic indicators and treatment selection. Otolaryngol Head Neck Surg 2014;150(4):610–7.

30. Kadakia S, Ducic Y, Marra D, et al. The role of elective superficial parotidectomy in the treatment of temporal region squamous cell carcinoma. Oral Maxillofac Surg 2016;20:143–7.

31. Ahmed MM, Moore BA, Schmalbach CE. Utility of head and neck cutaneous squamous cell carcinoma sentinel node biopsy: a systematic review. Otolaryngol Head Neck Surg 2014;150:180–7.

32. Veness M, Morgan GJ, Palme CE, et al. Surgery and adjuvant radiotherapy in patients with cutaneous head and neck squamous cell carcinoma metastatic to lymph nodes: combined treatment should be considered best practice. Laryngoscope 2015;115:870–5.

33. Mendenhall WM, Ferlito A, Takes RP, et al. Cutaneous head and neck basal and squamous cell carcinomas with perineural invasion. Oral Oncol 2012;48:918–22.

34. Bernier J, Domenge C, Ozsahin M, et al. Postoperative irradiation with or without concomitant chemotherapy for locally advanced head and neck cancer. N Engl J Med 2004;350:1945–52.

35. Chen F, Luo H, Xing L, et al. Feasibility and efficiency of concurrent chemoradiotherapy with capecitabine and cisplatin versus radiotherapy alone for elderly patients with locally advanced esophageal squamous cell carcinoma: experience of two centers. Thorac Cancer 2018;9(1):59–65.

36. Maubec E, Petrow P, Scheer-Senyarich I, et al. Phase II study of cetuximab as first-line single-drug therapy in patients with unresectable squamous cell carcinoma of the skin. J Clin Oncol 2011;29(25):3419–26.

37. Lewis CM, Glisson BS, Feng L, et al. A phase II study of gefitinib for aggressive cutaneous squamous cell carcinoma of the head and neck. Clin Cancer Res 2012;18(5):1435–46.

38. Tran DC, Coleva AD, Chang ALS. Follow-up on programmed cell death 1 inhibitor for cutaneous squamous cell carcinoma. JAMA Dermatol 2017;153:92–4.

39. Toker C. Trabecular carcinoma of the skin. Arch Dermatol 1972;105:107–10.

40. Dinh V, Feun L, Elgart G, et al. Merkel cell carcinomas. Hematol Oncol Clin North Am 2007;21:527–44.

41. Hodgson NC. Merkel cell carcinoma: changing incidence trends. J Surg Oncol 2005;89:1–4.

42. Padgett JK. Cutaneous lesions: benign and malignant. Facial Plast Surg Clin North Am 2005;13:195–202.

43. Miller NJ, Church CD, Dong L, et al. Tumor-infiltrating Merkel cell polyomavirus specific T cells are diverse and associated with improved patient survival. Cancer Immunol Res 2017;5:137–47.

44. Bichakjian CK, Olencki T, Andersen AM, et al. Merkel cell carcinoma, version 1.2014. J Natl Compr Canc Netw 2014;12:410–24.

45. Heath M, Jaimes N, Lemos B, et al. Clinical characteristics of Merkel cell carcinoma at diagnosis in 195 patients: the AEIOU features. J Am Acad Dermatol 2008;58:375–81.

46. Schmalbach CE, Lowe L, Teknos TN, et al. Reliability of sentinel lymph node biopsy for regional staging of head and neck Merkel cell carcinoma. Arch Otolaryngol Head Neck Surg 2005;131:610–4.

47. National Comprehensive Cancer Network clinical practice guidelines in oncology: Merkel cell carcinoma; version I.2018. 2017.

48. McGuire JF, Ge NN, Dyson S. Nonmelanoma skin cancer of the head and neck I: histopathology and clinical behavior. Am J Otolaryngol 2009;30:121–33.

49. Miles BA, Goldenberg D. Merkel cell carcinoma: do you know your guidelines? Head Neck 2016;38:647–52.

50. Veness MJ, Palme CE, Morgan GJ. Merkel cell carcinoma: a review of management. Curr Opin Otolaryngol Head Neck Surg 2008;16:170–4.

51. Tai P, Yu E, Assouline A, et al. Multimodality management for 145 cases of Merkel cell carcinoma. Med Oncol 2010;27:1260–6.

52. American Cancer Society. Cancer facts & figures 2016. Atlanta (GA): American Cancer Society; 2016.

53. American Academy of Dermatology. Melanoma/skin cancer: you can recognize the signs. In: American Academy of Dermatology, editor. AAD patient handout. Evanston (IL): 1986. Available at: https://www.aad.org/members/patient-education. Accessed November 12, 2017.

54. Abbasi NR, Shaw HM, Rigel DS, et al. Early diagnosis of cutaneous melanoma: revisiting the ABCD criteria. JAMA 2004;292:2771–6.

55. Prieto VG, Argenyi ZB, Barnhil RL, et al. Are en face frozen sections accurate for diagnosing margin status in melanocytic lesions? Am J Clin Pathol 2003;120: 203–8.

56. Zenga J, Nussenbaum B, Cornelius LA, et al. Management controversies in head and neck melanoma: a systematic review. JAMA Facial Plast Surg 2017;19: 53–62.

57. National Comprehensive Cancer Network clinical practice guidelines in oncology: Melanoma; version I.2017. 2016.

58. Schmalbach CE, Bradford CR. Is sentinel lymph node biopsy the standard of care for cutaneous head and neck melanoma? Laryngoscope 2015;125:153–60.

59. Durham AB, Schwartz JL, Lowe L, et al. The natural history of thin melanoma and the utility of sentinel lymph node biopsy. J Surg Oncol 2017;116(8):1185–92.

60. Faries MB, Thompson JF, Cochran AJ, et al. Completion dissection or observation for sentinel node metastasis in melanoma. N Engl J Med 2017;376:2211–22.

61. Mocellin S, Lens MB, Pasquali S, et al. Interferon alpha for the adjuvant treatment of cutaneous melanoma. Cochrane Database Syst Rev 2013;(6):CD008955.

62. Lasithiotakis KG, Petrakis IE, Garbe C. Cutaneous melanoma in the elderly: epidemiology, prognosis, and treatment. Melanoma Res 2010;20:163–70.

63. Robert C, Long GV, Brady B, et al. Nivolumab in previously untreated melanoma without BRAF mutation. N Engl J Med 2015;372:320–30.

64. Lemech C, Infante J, Arkenau HT. The potential for BRAF V600 inhibitors in advanced cutaneous melanoma: rationale and latest evidence. Ther Adv Med Oncol 2012;4:61–73.

Thyroid Disorders in the Elderly: An Overall Summary

Kevin Higgins, MD, MSc, FRCSC

KEYWORDS

- Elderly • Thyroid nodules • Cancer • Thyroid biochemistry

KEY POINTS

- Thyroid nodules are very common, and the workup should be tailored to risk.
- Thyroid cancer in the elderly tends to be more aggressive and surgery risk is greater based on performance status, and physiologic, not chronologic age.
- Thyroid biochemical abnormalities in the elderly are common, and can be mistakenly attributed to the normal process of aging.

INTRODUCTION

In 2013, there were 44.7 million people over the age of 65 in the United States and current projections suggest this number will more than double to 98 million by 2060.[1] Similarly, in 2003, 3.3% of North Americans were over the age of 79. This cohort is expected to increase to 5.3% by 2030.[2] As a result of decreasing fertility and increasing longevity, in a growing number of countries, one-half of the world's population will be accounted for by those aged 60 and over.

Thyroid disease in the elderly can be classified as functional disorders (hypothyroidism and hyperthyroidism), inflammatory conditions (thyroiditis), and neoplastic conditions (nodules and carcinomas). The prevalence of these conditions has been shown to increase with age.

Ninety percent of women present with thyroid nodules after the age of 60, and 60% of men present after the age of 80.[3] Almost 50% of patients greater than 65 years of age demonstrate nodules, on ultrasound scan. Similar prevalence has been found among autopsies performed in the general population.[4,5]

ANATOMIC AND PHYSIOLOGIC CHANGES

Postmortem examination of individuals aged 50 or older confirmed a decrease in gland volume with age. Progressive atrophy, fibrosis, and lymphocytic infiltration,

Disclosure Statement: There is no conflict of interest. The author declares no financial interests.
Department of Otolaryngology–Head and Neck Surgery, Sunnybrook Health Sciences Centre, 2075 Bayview Avenue, Toronto, Ontario M4N 3M5, Canada
E-mail address: kevin.higgins@sunnybrook.ca

Clin Geriatr Med 34 (2018) 259–277
https://doi.org/10.1016/j.cger.2018.01.011
0749-0690/18/© 2018 Elsevier Inc. All rights reserved.

geriatric.theclinics.com

with increased adipose tissue and decreased follicles and colloid, were implicated in this volume reduction.[6–8] The prevalence of autoantibodies increases with age, reaching up to 20% in women over 60 years of age and may be partly responsible for the observed anatomic changes in the thyroid gland as it ages.[9] This finding corroborates with previous reports suggesting that hypoechogenicity of the gland is linked to circulating antithyroid antibodies, reflecting inflammatory thyroiditis.[10,11]

The hypothalamic–pituitary–thyroid axis regulates thyroid synthesis, even in the elderly (**Fig. 1**). Iodine status in the elderly may be lower compared with young adults owing to dietary restrictions of salt, and decreased absorption owing to comorbid conditions or medicines.[9] Furthermore, thyroidal iodine uptake decreases with age. The net result is decreased thyroxine secretion in the elderly.[12] This reduction is compensated for however, by a decreased thyroxine metabolic clearance; 5'-deiodinase activity decreases with advancing age, which results in lower triiodothyronine levels.[12] Free hormone levels may remain stable with decreased thyroid binding globulin, whereas the inactive metabolite rT3 seems to increase with age. It is known that secretion of thyroid-stimulating hormone (TSH), in response to thyroid releasing hormone, is decreased in the elderly. This finding is possibly the result of insensitivity of thyroid cells in the anterior pituitary, and as explained by Bremner and colleagues,[13] an age-related alteration in the bioactivity of the TSH set point.[14] These alterations in the levels of hormones related to the pituitary–thyroid axis are associated with the process of aging and, as a result, may impact longevity. However, the direction of these changes still seems to be not fully determined.[15,16]

Thyroid cells are able to counteract potentially toxic expositions to reactive oxygen species (ROS) thanks to a fine-tuned antioxidant system. However, excess ROS production and/or inadequate production of antioxidants during aging, may contribute to oxidative stress and thyroid damage, including thyroidal autoimmune disease and cancer.[17,18] Additionally, thyroid hormones are known to accelerate metabolism and increase oxygen consumption. This condition leads to increased ROS, oxidative stress, and an acceleration in the basal metabolic rate.[19,20] Thyroid hormones are able to unsaturate membrane lipids, leading to membrane damage. This damage is most often exhibited in heart, spleen, and muscle tissues.[21] Recently, it has been demonstrated that binding of triiodothyronine to thyroid hormone receptor beta induces DNA damage and cell senescence. Hypothyroidism was found to be associated with reduced ROS generation and oxidative damage, whereas hyperthyroidism increased ROS production.[22,23] A slightly lower thyroid function, and thus a lower basal metabolic rate, could possibly serve as an adaptive mechanism to rule out excessive metabolism in the elderly. Thus, an increase in TSH seems to play a favorable role in health status.[24]

BIOCHEMISTRY: OVERT HYPOTHYROIDISM AND HYPERTHYROIDISM

Longevity is a complex multifactorial phenomenon where specific biological assets, such as hormonal networks, are impacted. Overt hypothyroidism occurs in 2% to 5% of patients older than 60 years.[16,25] Experimental evidence suggests that the hypothyroid state may favor longevity by reducing the metabolic rate, oxidative stress, and cell senescence. Although human studies seem to confirm this view, thyroid hormone changes observed in older patients cannot always be interpreted as a protective-adaptive mechanism. In some instances, medications interfere with thyroid function and their impact on these mechanisms is yet to be elucidated.[24]

A 20-year follow-up survey showed a positive correlation between age and incidence of increased antithyroid antibodies and hypothyroidism.[25] Recent National

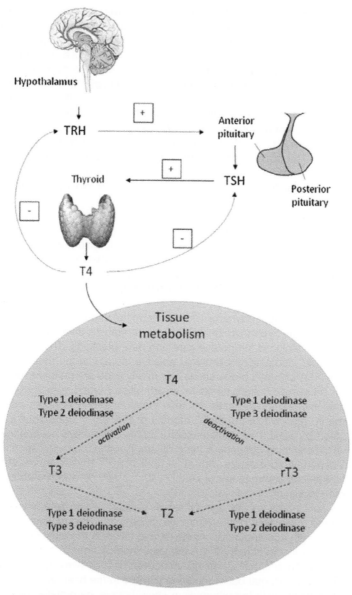

Fig. 1. The hypothalamic pituitary thyroid axis and peripheral metabolism of thyroid hormones. TRH, thyrotropin-releasing hormone; TSH, thyroid-stimulating hormone. (*From* Garasto S, Montesanto A, Corsonello A, et al. Thyroid hormones in extreme longevity. Mech Aging Dev 2017;165(Pt B):98–106; with permission.)

Health and Nutrition Examination Survey III surveys showed that serum TSH concentration, serum thyroid peroxidase, and thyroglobulin antibodies increase with age in both genders.[26] The cardiovascular system in the elderly retains its sensitivity to thyroid hormone action. As an example, atrial fibrillation with a slow ventricular rate is seen in up to 20% of elderly hyperthyroid patients. Other implicated associations include an adverse lipid profile, increased carotid intimal thickness, and endothelial dysfunction.[27,28] Biochemical abnormalities, particularly in patients with preexisting cardiac conditions, exhibited stronger association with significant cardiac morbidity and mortality in the elderly. Thyroid function tests require careful examination as reference ranges must be age adjusted and polypharmacy must be considered.

There are fewer studies that report the prevalence of hyperthyroidism. Estimates in elderly populations range from 0.5% to 5.8%, although typically they decrease around 1.5% in women and 1.0% in men over the age of 60.[12,16,29] Grave's disease is the most common cause of hyperthyroidism in all age groups (50%–70%). Multinodular goiter (30%–40%) increases with old age and is more frequent in geographic locations with adequate iodine intake.[16,30] Hyperthyroidism, owing to thyroiditis, constitutes less than 5% of the elderly population. Iodine-induced thyrotoxicosis is more prevalent in the elderly owing to radiocontrast agents and iodine moieties contained in amiodarone or mucolytics.[16,30]

Hyperthyroidism is a diagnostic challenge in the elderly because of its atypical presentation. Despite the classic list of symptoms often exhibited by younger patients with hyperthyroidism (tremor, weight loss, palpitations, diarrhea, and heat intolerance), elderly patients may present asymptomatically. When agitation and confusion constitute the symptoms, the potential cause is termed "=apathetic toxicosis.[31] Graves' ophthalmopathy is seen less frequently, but, when present, is more severe and difficult to manage.[30,32]

The management of hyperthyroidism depends on the underlying mechanism. It can be related to subacute hyperthyroidism or silent lymphocytic thyroiditis. The management of thyroiditis includes supportive care and beta-blockade. Therapeutic options include antithyroid medications or thyroid ablative therapy in the form of surgery or iodine therapy.[33] Antithyroid medications commonly used are methimazole and propylthiouracil. These medications cause fever, arthralgias, or a rash in 1% to 5% of patients. Agranulocytosis and hepatitis are seen more commonly in elderly patients and most commonly seen within the first 3 months of therapy.[34] Beta-blockade can be contraindicated by patient morbidities such chronic obstructive pulmonary disease or asthma and coexisting congestive heart failure. Routine anticoagulation is recommended in hyperthyroid patients with atrial fibrillation.[35] Thyroid storm and severe thyrotoxicosis is less common in the elderly with surgery, and iodine ablation is the most common trigger.[36]

Hypothyroidism increases with age. Of elderly patients, 7% to 14% have some TSH levels above the upper limit of the reference ranges.[26,37] The presence of autoantibodies increase with age and autoimmune thyroid failure is the most common cause of hypothyroidism in the elderly.[38,39] Antibodies include antimicrosomal antibodies and antithyroglobulin antibodies. Iatrogenic causes of hypothyroidism include drugs such as lithium and external beam radiation therapy in the head and neck region.[12] Some elderly patients with hypothyroidism show fatigue, mental slowness, drowsiness, depression, constipation, heat intolerance, and weight gain. Symptoms related to hypothyroidism are often incorrectly attributed to normal age-related changes. It must be stressed, in these instances, that the patient's cognitive decline and delirium are due to hypothyroidism and are, therefore, potentially reversible. Hypothyroidism can also present with cerebellar dysfunction and anemia, as well as voice changes, such as Reinke's edema.[40,41] Elderly hypothyroid patients are more sensitive to large, corrective thyroid hormone replacement dosing. Extended incidences of excess thyroid hormone can cause cardiac arrhythmias and angina. The initial dose, for patients without cardiac morbidity, is 25 µg/d. For patients with cardiac comorbidities, the initial dose is 12.5 µg/d. Once the tolerance and safety profile is confirmed, most experts increase doses by 12.5 to 25.0 µg every 4 weeks until TSH values gradually normalize. In most carefully controlled studies, one of the parameters spontaneously returns to normal in about 25% to 50% of patients.[42,43]

THYROID NODULES: DIAGNOSIS, WORKUP, AND MANAGEMENT

It is estimated that nodular thyroid disease affects about 90% of females 60 years of age and older and 60% of males 80 years of age and older.[3,4] Of these, 5% harbor a malignant lesion in the adult population.[44,45] Prospective studies show that 13% to 28% of thyroid (colloid) nodules can shrink over a 2- to 3-year period and may disappear in 22% of patients.[46] After ionizing radiation, the incidence of new nodules increases at the rate of 2% per year and reaches a peak incidence after 15 to 25 years.[47]

Fine needle aspiration cytology represents the main diagnostic tool for the evaluation of nodules and suspicious cervical lymph nodes.[48] Fine needle aspiration biopsy of thyroid nodules shows a sensitivity of 65% to 98%, a specificity of 72% to 100%, and an accuracy of 84% to 95%.[49,50] The Bethesda system (**Fig. 2**) for reporting thyroid cytopathology lists cytologic categorization as follows: 1, nondiagnostic; 2, benign; 3, atypia/follicular lesion of indeterminate significance; 4, follicular neoplasm or suspicious for follicular neoplasm; 5, suspicious for malignancy; and 6, malignant.[51,52] Although fine-needle aspiration cytology diagnosis is very reliable, diagnostic categories 3 to 5 present a gray zone.[49,52] The accuracy of fine-needle aspiration cytology depends on the experience and skill of the cytopathologist.[53,54] Inadequate cellularity in nonrepresentative samples account for about 20% of specimens.[55,56] However, the prognosis is generally favorable with 10-year survival for well-differentiated thyroid cancer at about 90%.[57,58]

In 1 study, when cytologic results were compared individually, malignant cytology was higher (32.5% vs 22.0%) and nondiagnostic cytology was lower (9%) in geriatric patients. This finding did not reach statistical significance, however ($P = .068$).[59]

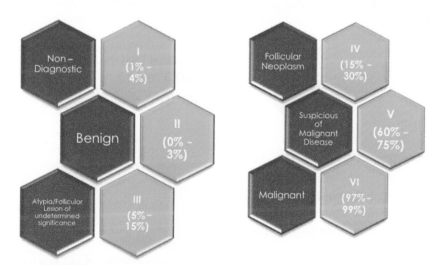

Fig. 2. Thyroid nodule evaluation: Bethesda system. (*Data from* Tuttle M. Long term follow-up and surveillance of thyroid cancer - using response to therapy assessments to guide follow-up recommendations. 2013. Available at: http://thyroidworldcongress.com/wp-content/uploads/2013/07/5-Long-term-Follow-up-and-Surveillance-of-Thyroid-Cancer-R.-Michael-Tuttle.pdf. Accessed February 1, 2017.)

Ultrasound features predictable for malignancy seem to not differ in elderly and younger patients.[59] Based on the revised American Thyroid Association 2015 guidelines, cytologic sampling should be considered for the indications in **Figs. 3** and **4**, with the important caveat that TSH levels should be measured before needle biopsy.[57]

THYROID CANCER SURGERY AND CARE PATHWAY (DEESCALATION AND EMERGING ACTIVE SURVEILLANCE)
Thyroid Cancer (Epidemiology)

In older adults, differentiated thyroid cancers are more advanced, and mortality and recurrence rates are higher.[60,61] More aggressive histopathologic patterns, poor general physical condition, and delayed diagnosis are potential reasons to explain this worse prognosis.[62,63]

Thyroid cancer is the most common malignancy in the endocrine system, constituting 2% of all malignancies. Papillary thyroid cancer (PTC) is the common pathologic type; it accounts for 90% of thyroid cancers. PTC has almost a bell-shaped distribution of age at presentation, with 60% of patients presenting at 30 to 59 years of age (**Fig. 5**).[64] Gender, age, tumor size, extrathyroidal extension, node status, and metastases are well-established prognostic factors for PTC.[65,66] Between 1973 and 2002, the incidence of thyroid cancer increased approximately 240% from 3.6 to 8.7 per 100,000 person population, although disease-specific mortality rate remains largely stable (pegged at 0.5 deaths per 100,000),[67] this increase in prevalence has been attributed to improved imaging methods in higher sensitivity ultrasound; there are also studies that suggest a real increase.[68,69]

Mazzaferri and Kloos and their colleagues[70,71] concluded that the risk of death owing to thyroid cancer gradually increases with each subsequent year of life and then dramatically escalates after age 60. Thyroid staging remains unique in the inclusion of age in the TNM guidelines with the widely recommended age cut at 45 to 55,

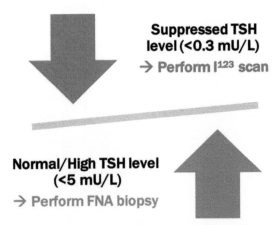

Suppressed TSH level (<0.3 mU/L)
→ Perform I¹²³ scan

Normal/High TSH level (<5 mU/L)
→ Perform FNA biopsy

Fig. 3. The American Thyroid Association (ATA) recommends serum thyroid-stimulating hormone (TSH) measurement and neck ultrasonography in all patients with a thyroid nodule. FNA, fine needle aspiration. (*Data from* Haugen BR, Alexander EK, Bible KC, et al. 2015 American Thyroid Association management guidelines for adult patients with thyroid nodules and differentiated thyroid cancer: the American Thyroid Association Guidelines Task Force on thyroid nodules and differentiated thyroid cancer. Thyroid 2016;26:1–133.)

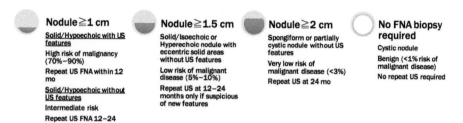

Nodule≥1 cm	Nodule≥1.5 cm	Nodule≥2 cm	No FNA biopsy required
Solid/Hypoechoic with US features	Solid/Isoechoic or Hyperechoic nodule with eccentric solid areas without US features	Spongiform or partially cystic nodule without US features	Cystic nodule
High risk of malignancy (70%–90%)	Low risk of malignant disease (5%–10%)	Very low risk of malignant disease (<3%)	Benign (<1% risk of malignant disease)
Repeat US FNA within 12 mo	Repeat US at 12–24 months only if suspicious of new features	Repeat US at 24 mo	No repeat US required
Solid/Hypoechoic without US features			
Intermediate risk			
Repeat US FNA 12–24 mo			

Fig. 4. American Thyroid Association (ATA) recommended timeline for repeat ultrasound as a function of nodule features. FNA, fine needle aspiration; US, ultrasound. (*Data from* Haugen BR, Alexander EK, Bible KC, et al. 2015 American Thyroid Association management guidelines for adult patients with thyroid nodules and differentiated thyroid cancer: the American Thyroid Association Guidelines Task Force on thyroid nodules and differentiated thyroid cancer. Thyroid 2016;26(1):1–133.)

resulting in advanced staging.[72,73] However, there is a remarkably different pattern of tumor recurrence, which is greatest at the extremes of life—before age 20 and after age 60—with a recurrence rate of 40%.[74] The incidence of differentiated thyroid cancer increases steeply then plateaus at age 65 to 69.[75] After 69 years of age, the incidence of thyroid cancer steeply declines.

A study examining the aggressiveness of thyroid cancer in the elderly states that 70% had locally advanced disease, 44% had advanced nodal disease, and 23% had distant metastasis.[76] Park and associates[77] showed that patients 65 years or older exhibited a more aggressive disease course, with multiple, large tumors, more nonpapillary histology, and extrathyroidal extension. In support, larger tumors are notable in the elderly, which may result from delayed diagnosis and aggressive behavior.[60,77] Well-differentiated carcinomas, such as sclerosing and tall cell, were reported to be more frequent in older ages.[61,78] Hurthle cell cancer is one example with a

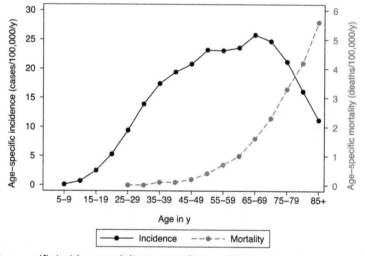

Fig. 5. Age-specific incidence and disease-specific mortality for thyroid cancer in the United States, 2007 to 2011. (*From* McLeod DSA, Carruthers K, Kevat DAS. Optimal differentiated thyroid cancer management in the elderly. Drugs Aging 2015;32(4):283–94.)

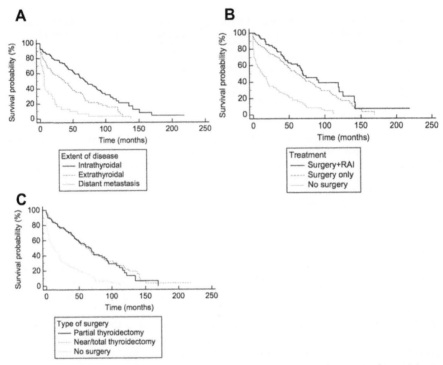

Fig. 6. Kaplan-Meier survival curves according to extent of disease (*A; P < .001*), participants with surgery versus no surgery (*B; P < .001*), and type of surgery (*C; P = .92*). RAI, radioactive iodine. (*From* Marvin K, Parham K. Differentiated thyroid cancer in people aged 85 and older. J Am Geriatr Soc 2015;63(5):935; with permission.)

higher metastatic potential within the well-differentiated thyroid cancers in the elderly[79] (**Fig. 6**).

The 10-year relative survival for individuals with PTC has been reported at 99% for patients younger than 20 years of age and 86% for patients greater than 70 years of age. Population-based studies using the National Cancer Institute/Surveillance, Epidemiology, and End Results database found that 2.7% of patients with thyroid cancer as the malignancy ultimately died of their disease. With those aged 75 and older, the 5-year incidence of death was 12.2%. The overall mortality from thyroid cancer was 3.53%, but the relative percentage breakdown of mortality was 22.5% in the geriatric population and 0.89% in the nongeriatric patient population[80] (**Fig. 7**).

Age at diagnosis was an independent prognostic factor in several large retrospective series. The report from Vini and colleagues[76] demonstrated that, with any 10-year difference in age, there was near doubling of the risk for recurrence, and that death increases linearly with age. A higher prevalence of biological risk factors like vascular invasion, extracapsular extension, and follicular type is more common in older patients.[3,61,62,77] Vini and colleagues[76] continued to report that the median time from therapy to clinical recurrence for well-differentiated thyroid cancer was only 9 months for the elderly group, compared with an average of 34 months in the whole series of 1390 adults. In geriatric and nongeriatric groups, 2.0% and 0.2% of tumors were anaplastic, respectively, which is a statistically significant difference.[59]

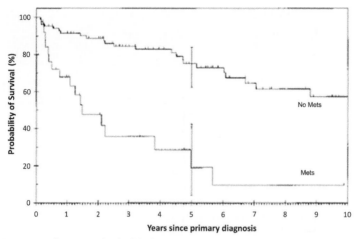

Fig. 7. Cause-specific survival of elderly patients with differentiated thyroid carcinoma comparing patients who developed metastases (Mets) with patients who did not develop metastases (No Mets). (*From* Matsuyama H, Sugitani I, Fujimoto Y, et al. Indications for thyroid cancer surgery in elderly patients. Surg Today 2009;39(8):652–7; with permission.)

Ito and colleagues[81] studied papillary microcancers for decades and found that only 8% of observed microcancers showed significant growth within 10 years. This finding suggests that initiation of papillary microcancers was not in adults, but young children.[81] All papillary microcancers in young patients grew faster compared with older patients (>60 years of age), who had no observable growth. Further, not a single patient among the 1235 died from thyroid cancer in this observation trial.[81] Considering that 10% of patients die from thyroid cancer in general,[82,83] it is unlikely that these PMCs show progression to lethal cancers.[84] Elderly patients generally show worse disease-specific survival as opposed to middle-aged or young adults. Young patients with PTC show higher recurrence rates, yet excellent survival. These confusing age-related epiphenomena are not well-explained.[70,85,86] An emerging theory concerning thyroid carcinogenesis that seems to explain this observed bimodal biologic behavior is that immature cancers remain silent for decades and start proliferation after middle age. Owing to their capacity to proliferate, they are associated with a poor prognosis and can be lethal. Mature and immature cancers can look pathologically similar, but are different in the origin, growth, and clinical course. The growth rate and thyroglobulin doubling time is the surrogate marker of this malignant potential. This frame shift in our understanding of thyroid cancer aggressiveness has led to a deescalation of initial thyroid disease management (**Fig. 8**).

SPECIFIC CONSIDERATIONS IN THE ELDERLY: POSTOPERATIVE THYROID-STIMULATING HORMONE SUPPRESSION

Current American Thyroid Association guidelines[57] and National Comprehensive Cancer Network Clinical Practice Guidelines[87] both recommend controlling postoperative serum TSH at values at lower than 0.1 in moderate- to high-risk patients with PTC, and 0.1 to 0.5 in intermediate-risk patients. The most recent published analysis of the National Comprehensive Cancer Network study found that patients with stage 3 or 4

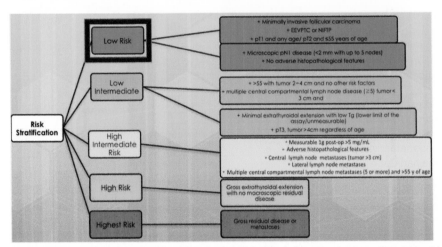

Fig. 8. Risk stratification pathway. EECPTC, entirely encapsulated variant papillary thyroid cancer; NIFTP, noninvasive follicular thyroid neoplasm with papillary-like nuclear features; Tg, thyroglobulin. (*Data from* Haugen BR, Alexander EK, Bible KC, et al. 2015 American Thyroid Association management guidelines for adult patients with thyroid nodules and differentiated thyroid cancer: the American Thyroid Association Guidelines Task Force on thyroid nodules and differentiated thyroid cancer. Thyroid 2016;26:1–133; and Thyroid cancer pathway map. Cancer Care Ontario; 2017. Available at: https://www.cancercareontario.ca/en/pathway-maps/thyroid-cancer. Accessed January 17, 2018.)

disease who had suppressed serum TSH during follow-up seemed to have a better overall disease-specific survival.[88] Patients with stage 2 disease seemed to have a better prognosis if TSH values were not increased. Patients with stage 1 disease had an excellent prognosis regardless of the TSH at follow-up.[88] In patients who are older, the risks of suppressive therapy seems to outweigh the potential benefits and a TSH target in the lower part of the normal range (0.5–2.0) is more reasonable.[89] This is because patient's age and cardiac function must also be considered to avoid effects of cardiotoxicity and osteoporosis.[90] Additional consideration must also be paid to pharmacodynamics and pharmacokinetics in the elderly.

Even though elderly patients have more severe disease, they are more prone to complications after postoperative endocrine therapy.[90] A 5-year follow-up study revealed significant differences in development of arrhythmias and osteoporosis, insomnia and anxiety between groups with differential suppression levels: B (TSH 0.1–0.3 MIU/mL) and C (TSH < 0.1 MIU/mL) compared with group A (0.3–0.5 MIU/mL).[90]

ADJUVANT THERAPY: RADIOACTIVE IODINE, EXTERNAL BEAM RADIATION, AND CHEMOTHERAPY

Radioactive iodine (RAI) is a targeted radioisotope therapy that is directed at follicular-derived thyroid cells, which take up iodine via the sodium–iodine transporter. These thyroid cells then trap and organify the iodine.[91] The RAI emits beta particles to damage and ultimately destroy adjacent thyroid tissue. RAI is usually well-tolerated and adverse affects are uncommon.[91]

The role of adjuvant RAI improves survival by an average of 9 months for patients at high risk; however, this difference is not statistically significant. It is generally thought that RAI decreases locoregional recurrence as opposed to affecting disease-specific mortality. Side effects include gastritis, sialadenitis, xerostomia, bone marrow suppression, pneumonitis, and dacryocystitis. High doses of RAI require hospital admission and confinement usually for 72 hours. Further, a dose of 200 mCi could exceed the maximum dose for older patients.[92] Because older patients may require assistance with activities of daily life, the use of RAI may be limited. Two intramuscular injections of recombinant TSH, 72 hours in advance of RAI is strongly encouraged in the elderly (>70 years of age), given the marked sensitivity toward any prolonged 4-week hypothyroid state.[92]

Ronga and colleagues[93] found that almost all patients 45 years old or younger with lung metastasis had RAI uptake, whereas significantly fewer greater than 45 years of age had uptake within the metastatic focus. Thus, although thyroid cancer cells seem to be more morphologically differentiated with increased age, there may be shifts away from thyroid-specific cell expression. This finding indicates a less differentiated malignant phenotype in some patients, rendering administration less effective in the elderly.[70] Schlumberger and colleagues[94] noted I[131] uptake at metastatic sites in only 53% of patients older than 40 years of age, compared with 90% of patients younger than 40 years of age.

It has previously been shown that external beam radiation achieves local control in 81% of patients when residual microscopic disease is present and achieves local control in 37% of patients when macroscopic residual disease is present. Radiotherapy can be used as a form of palliation for distressing locoregional symptoms. Doses of 40 to 50 Gy to the thyroid bed are typically recommended when local invasion into trachea, carotid sheath, or esophagus precludes complete surgical extirpation. Late effects of external beam radiation include esophageal stricture, dysphasia, tracheotomy tube placement relating to laryngeal edema, or stenosis.[95] With the emergence of enhanced 3-dimensioanl conformal radiation delivery techniques, including intensity-modulated radiation therapy, there is less of a risk of complications resulting from collateral damage to critical structures.

The use of conventional chemotherapy such as doxorubicin has been discouraged by recent differentiated thyroid cancer guidelines.[57,96] However, phase II and III trials of tyrosine kinase inhibitors have emerged as possible treatment options for patients with metastatic or locally advanced differentiated thyroid cancer with no iodine uptake.[91] Sorafenib was the first kinase inhibitor approved for use in differentiated thyroid cancer, with recent approval from the US Food and Drug Administration for lenvatinib.[91] Sorafenib improved progression-free survival in phase III studies.[97] Common side effects include hand and foot desquamative skin rashes, alopecia, and serious issues, including colitis and pneumonitis.[98] One concern with kinas inhibitors is the potential for accelerated disease progression with treatment cessation and grade 5 toxicity.[99]

SURVEILLANCE AND MANAGEMENT OF RECURRENCE

Remission can be clinically defined as no clinical or radiologic evidence of tumor with a serum thyroglobulin levels of less than 2 ng/ML during TSH suppression and with stimulation in the absence of antithyroglobulin antibodies.[61,100] The overall response to therapy is summarized in **Fig. 9**.

After total thyroidectomy and RAI ablation, the reported risk of recurrence was 1% to 5% (median, 1.8%) over 5 to 10 years of follow-up. Patients reported as exhibiting a biochemically incomplete response demonstrate persistent abnormal thyroglobulin values in the absence of localizable disease. After 5 to 10 years of follow-up, 34%

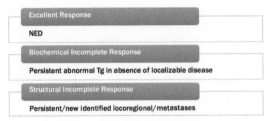

Fig. 9. Summary of the overall response to therapy. NED, no evidence of disease; Tg, thyroglobulin. (*Data from* Tuttle M. Long term follow-up and surveillance of thyroid cancer - using response to therapy assessments to guide follow-up recommendations. 2013. Available at: http://thyroidworldcongress.com/wp-content/uploads/2013/07/5-Long-term-Follow-up-and-Surveillance-of-Thyroid-Cancer-R.-Michael-Tuttle.pdf. Accessed February 1, 2017.)

of patients evolve to showing no evidence of disease with no additional therapy, 35% show no evidence of disease after additional treatments, and only 8% to 17% develop structural disease (almost always heralded by increasing thyroglobulin or thyroglobulin antibodies over time). There were no disease specific deaths in this subgroup (**Fig. 10**).

Finally, patients reported as having a structural incomplete response to therapy have persistent or newly identified locoregional or distant metastases. Despite additional treatments, the majority of these patients have persistent structural disease at the final follow-up. There is an 11% death rate associated with structural locoregional disease, and a 57% death rate with structural distant metastases, based on 5- to 10-year follow-up data, has been observed. American Thyroid Association guidelines in fact recommend biopsy of suspicious lymph nodes (including thyroid bed and lateral basin) with the smallest diameter (short axis) greater than 5 to 8 mm, if a positive result will ultimately change management.

The cornerstone of follow-up and discriminating biochemically persistent disease has been shown to be the thyroglobulin doubling time measured under TSH suppressed conditions. Thyroglobulin doubling time has emerged as a very potent

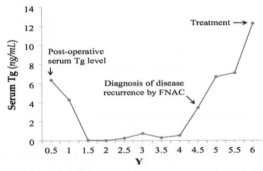

Fig. 10. Postoperative serum thyroglobulin (Tg) levels in the single study patient who developed recurrent disease during follow-up. FNAC, fine-needle aspiration cytology. (*From* Durante C, Montesano T, Attard M, et al. Long-term surveillance of papillary thyroid cancer patients who do not undergo postoperative radioiodine remnant ablation: is there a role for serum thyroglobulin measurement? J Clin Endocrinol Metab 2012;97(8):2752; with permission.)

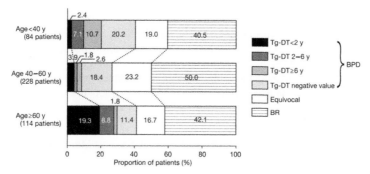

Fig. 11. Postoperative thyroglobulin status and thyroglobulin-doubling time (Tg-DT) according to age in 426 patients with papillary thyroid carcinoma (PTC) who underwent total thyroidectomy. (*From* Miyauchi A, Kudo T, Kihara M, et al. Relationship of biochemically persistent disease and thyroglobulin-doubling time to age at surgery in patients with papillary thyroid carcinoma. Endocr J 2013;60(4):417; with permission.)

prognostic indicator in patients with PTC. In a univariate analysis, only those greater than 60 years old with a hazard ratio of 6.72 remained significant. These results indicate that the tumor growth rate of hidden metastasis, as well as the thyroglobulin doubling time, is strongly related to age of patients at surgery.[101] Postoperatively, using data from 426 patients, 33% had biochemically persistent disease. The percentages were higher among the young (<40 years old) and elderly (≥60 years old) compared with middle-aged patients (40–60 years old). Multivariate analyses showed that lateral neck disease, with tumors greater than 4 cm and extrathyroidal extension, were significantly associated with biochemically persistent disease (**Fig. 11** and **Table 1**). Most tumors were slow growing or even possibly regressing, as indicated by the relatively long negative thyroglobulin doubling time values in patients within the present study cohort. All patients who died of disease had doubling time of less than 2, which is the key indicator of growth rate.[74]

Table 1
Multivariate analysis of factors that may be associated with thyroglobulin-doubling time shorter than 2 years in patients with biochemically persistent disease

Variables	Univariate Analysis			Multivariate Analysis		
	P value	Hazard Ratio	95% CI	P value	Hazard Ratio	95% CI
Male gender	.5202	0.71	0.24–2.04	—	—	—
Age ≥60 y	.0000	6.72	2.87–15.73	.0000	6.72	2.87–15.73
T ≥4 cm	.0681	2.13	0.95–4.81	—	—	—
Ex2	.0556	2.16	0.98–4.77	—	—	—
cN1b	.4909	0.75	0.34–1.68	—	—	—
M1	.8801	1.11	0.28–4.37	—	—	—

Abbreviations: CI, confidence interval; Ex2, significant extrathyroid extension, equivalent to pT4a in the TNM classification; T, tumor size.
From Miyauchi A, Kudo T, Kihara M, et al. Relationship of biochemically persistent disease and thyroglobulin-doubling time to age at surgery in patients with papillary thyroid carcinoma. Endocr J 2013;60(4):418; with permission.

SUMMARY

Age-related changes in thyroid biochemistry and anatomy are prevalent. Dysfunction can present atypically and should always be considered in dementia and delirium workups. Thyroid nodules and malignancy should be managed with an evidence-based approach recognizing the usefulness of surveillance while at the same time acknowledging the possibility of aggressiveness in this population.

ACKNOWLEDGMENTS

Article edited by Sabrina Rashid, Michael Hong, BSc, and Mario Orsini.

REFERENCES

1. Colby SL, Ortman JM. Projections of the size and composition of the U.S. population: 2014 to 2060, current population reports, P25-1143. Washington, DC: U.S. Census Bureau; 2014. p. 1–13. Available at: https://www.census.gov/content/dam/Census/library/publications/2015/demo/p25-1143.pdf. Accessed October 24, 2017.
2. Beahrs OH. Surgery of thyroid and parathyroid disorders in the aged. In: Adkins RB, Scott HW, editors. Surgical care for the elderly. Baltimore (MD): Williams & Wilkins; 1988. p. 128–37. Available at: https://www.researchgate.net/publication/242587560_Complications_of_thyroid_surgery_in_octogenarians_are_more_likely_caused_by_comorbidities_than_by_age_alone. Accessed March 9, 2018.
3. Gervasi R, Orlando G, Lerose MA, et al. Thyroid surgery in geriatric patients: a literature review. BMC Surg 2012;12(Suppl 1):S16.
4. Mekel M, Stephen AE, Gaz RD, et al. Thyroid surgery in octogenarians is associated with higher complication rates. Surgery 2009;146(5):913–21.
5. Seybt MW, Khichi S, Terris DJ. Geriatric thyroidectomy: safety of thyroid surgery in an aging population. Arch Otolaryngol Head Neck Surg 2009;135(10):1041–4.
6. Nafisi Moghadam R, Shajari A, Afkhami-Ardekani M. Influence of physiological factors on thyroid size determined by ultrasound. Acta Med Iran 2011;49(5):302–4.
7. Zou Y, Ding G, Lou X, et al. Factors influencing thyroid volume in Chinese children. Eur J Clin Nutr 2013;67(11):1138–41.
8. Brown RA, Al-Moussa M, Beck J. Histometry of normal thyroid in man. J Clin Pathol 1986;39(5):475–82.
9. Irvine RE. Thyroid disease in old age. In: Brock Lehurst JC, editor. Text book of pediatric medicine and gerontology. New York: Churchill Livingstone; 1973. p. 435–58.
10. Miranda DMC, Massom JN, Catarino RM, et al. Impact of nutritional iodine optimization on rates of thyroid hypoechogenicity and autoimmune thyroiditis: a cross-sectional, comparative study. Thyroid 2015;25(1):118–24.
11. Willms A, Bieler D, Wieler H, et al. Correlation between sonography and antibody activity in patients with Hashimoto thyroiditis. J Ultrasound Med 2013;32(11):1979–86.
12. Ajish TP, Jayakumar RV. Geriatric thyroidology: an update. Indian J Endocrinol Metab 2012;16(4):542–7.
13. Bremner AP, Feddema P, Leedman PJ, et al. Age-related changes in thyroid function: a longitudinal study of a community-based cohort. J Clin Endocrinol Metab 2012;97(5):1554–62.
14. Gesing A, Lewiński A, Karbownik-Lewińska M. The thyroid gland and the process of aging; what is new? Thyroid Res 2012;5(1):16.

15. Yeap BB. Hormones and health outcomes in aging men. Exp Gerontol 2013; 48(7):677–81.
16. Mariotti S, Franceschi C, Cossarizza A, et al. The aging thyroid. Endocr Rev 1995;16(6):686–715.
17. Burek CL, Rose NR. Autoimmune thyroiditis and ROS. Autoimmun Rev 2008; 7(7):530–7.
18. Vitale G, Salvioli S, Franceschi C. Oxidative stress and the ageing endocrine system. Nat Rev Endocrinol 2013;9(4):228–40.
19. Bangur CS, Howland JL, Katyare SS. Thyroid hormone treatment alters phospholipid composition and membrane fluidity of rat brain mitochondria. Biochem J 1995;305(Pt 1):29–32.
20. Gredilla R, López Torres M, Portero-Otín M, et al. Influence of hyper- and hypothyroidism on lipid peroxidation, unsaturation of phospholipids, glutathione system and oxidative damage to nuclear and mitochondrial DNA in mice skeletal muscle. Mol Cell Biochem 2001;221(1–2):41–8.
21. Villanueva I, Alva-Sánchez C, Pacheco-Rosado J. The role of thyroid hormones as inductors of oxidative stress and neurodegeneration. Oxid Med Cell Longev 2013;2013:218145.
22. Asayama K, Dobashi K, Hayashibe H, et al. Lipid peroxidation and free radical scavengers in thyroid dysfunction in the rat: a possible mechanism of injury to heart and skeletal muscle in hyperthyroidism. Endocrinology 1987;121(6):2112–8.
23. Yavuz DG, Yüksel M, Deyneli O, et al. Association of serum paraoxonase activity with insulin sensitivity and oxidative stress in hyperthyroid and TSH-suppressed nodular goitre patients. Clin Endocrinol (Oxf) 2004;61(4):515–21.
24. Garasto S, Montesanto A, Corsonello A, et al. Thyroid hormones in extreme longevity. Mech Ageing Dev 2017;165(Pt B):98–106.
25. Vanderpump MP, Tunbridge WM, French JM, et al. The incidence of thyroid disorders in the community: a twenty-year follow-up of the Whickham survey. Clin Endocrinol (Oxf) 1995;43(1):55–68.
26. Hollowell JG, Staehling NW, Flanders WD, et al. Serum TSH, T(4), and thyroid antibodies in the United States population (1988 to 1994): National Health and Nutrition Examination Survey (NHANES III). J Clin Endocrinol Metab 2002; 87(2):489–99.
27. Monzani F, Caraccio N, Kozàkowà M, et al. Effect of levothyroxine replacement on lipid profile and intima-media thickness in subclinical hypothyroidism: a double-blind, placebo- controlled study. J Clin Endocrinol Metab 2004;89(5): 2099–106.
28. Razvi S, Ingoe L, Keeka G, et al. The beneficial effect of L-thyroxine on cardiovascular risk factors, endothelial function, and quality of life in subclinical hypothyroidism: randomized, crossover trial. J Clin Endocrinol Metab 2007;92(5): 1715–23.
29. Parle JV, Franklyn JA, Cross KW, et al. Prevalence and follow-up of abnormal thyrotrophin (TSH) concentrations in the elderly in the United Kingdom. Clin Endocrinol (Oxf) 1991;34(1):77–83.
30. Díez JJ. Hyperthyroidism in patients older than 55 years: an analysis of the etiology and management. Gerontology 2003;49(5):316–23.
31. Trivalle C, Doucet J, Chassagne P, et al. Differences in the signs and symptoms of hyperthyroidism in older and younger patients. J Am Geriatr Soc 1996;44(1): 50–3.
32. Kendler DL, Lippa J, Rootman J. The initial clinical characteristics of Graves' orbitopathy vary with age and sex. Arch Ophthalmol 1993;111(2):197–201.

33. Solomon B, Glinoer D, Lagasse R, et al. Current trends in the management of Graves' disease. J Clin Endocrinol Metab 1990;70(6):1518–24.
34. Tajiri J, Noguchi S. Antithyroid drug-induced agranulocytosis: special reference to normal white blood cell count agranulocytosis. Thyroid 2004;14(6):459–62.
35. Aronow WS. The heart and thyroid disease. Clin Geriatr Med 1995;11(2):219–29.
36. Marcocci C, Kahaly GJ, Krassas GE, et al. Selenium and the course of mild Graves' orbitopathy. N Engl J Med 2011;364(20):1920–31.
37. Tunbridge WM, Evered DC, Hall R, et al. The spectrum of thyroid disease in a community: the Whickham survey. Clin Endocrinol (Oxf) 1977;7(6):481–93.
38. Mariotti S, Chiovato L, Franceschi C, et al. Thyroid autoimmunity and aging. Exp Gerontol 1998;33(6):535–41.
39. Pinchera A, Mariotti S, Barbesino G, et al. Thyroid autoimmunity and ageing. Horm Res 1995;43(1–3):64–8.
40. Mokshagundam S, Barzel US. Thyroid disease in the elderly. J Am Geriatr Soc 1993;41(12):1361–9.
41. Tachman ML, Guthrie GP. Hypothyroidism: diversity of presentation. Endocr Rev 1984;5(3):456–65.
42. Surks MI, Ortiz E, Daniels GH, et al. Subclinical thyroid disease: scientific review and guidelines for diagnosis and management. JAMA 2004;291(2):228–38.
43. Hegedüs L. Clinical practice. The thyroid nodule. N Engl J Med 2004;351(17):1764–71.
44. Welker MJ, Orlov D. Thyroid nodules. Am Fam Physician 2003;67(3):559–66.
45. Wang C-CC, Friedman L, Kennedy GC, et al. A large multicenter correlation study of thyroid nodule cytopathology and histopathology. Thyroid 2011;21(3):243–51.
46. Mazzaferri EL. Management of a solitary thyroid nodule. N Engl J Med 1993;328(8):553–9.
47. Zenilman ME. Surgery in the elderly. Curr Probl Surg 1998;35(2):99–179.
48. Sorrenti S, Baldini E, Tartaglia F, et al. Nodular thyroid disease in the elderly: novel molecular approaches for the diagnosis of malignancy. Aging Clin Exp Res 2017;29(Suppl 1):7–13.
49. Gharib H. Fine-needle aspiration biopsy of thyroid nodules: advantages, limitations, and effect. Mayo Clin Proc 1994;69(1):44–9.
50. Baloch ZW, Sack MJ, Yu GH, et al. Fine-needle aspiration of thyroid: an institutional experience. Thyroid 1998;8(7):565–9.
51. Cibas ES, Ali SZ, NCI Thyroid FNA State of the Science Conference. The Bethesda system for reporting thyroid cytopathology. Am J Clin Pathol 2009;132(5):658–65.
52. Baloch ZW, LiVolsi VA, Asa SL, et al. Diagnostic terminology and morphologic criteria for cytologic diagnosis of thyroid lesions: a synopsis of the National Cancer Institute Thyroid Fine-Needle Aspiration State of the Science Conference. Diagn Cytopathol 2008;36(6):425–37.
53. Florentine BD, Staymates B, Rabadi M, et al, Cancer Committee of the Henry Mayo Newhall Memorial Hospital. The reliability of fine-needle aspiration biopsy as the initial diagnostic procedure for palpable masses: a 4-year experience of 730 patients from a community hospital-based outpatient aspiration biopsy clinic. Cancer 2006;107(2):406–16.
54. Cignarelli M, Triggiani V, Ciampolillo A, et al. High frequency of incidental diagnosis of extrathyroidal neoplastic diseases at the fine-needle aspiration biopsy of laterocervical lymph nodes in patients with thyroid nodules. Thyroid 2001;11(1):65–71.

55. Ustün M, Risberg B, Davidson B, et al. Cystic change in metastatic lymph nodes: a common diagnostic pitfall in fine-needle aspiration cytology. Diagn Cytopathol 2002;27(6):387–92.
56. Kessler A, Rappaport Y, Blank A, et al. Cystic appearance of cervical lymph nodes is characteristic of metastatic papillary thyroid carcinoma. J Clin Ultrasound 2003;31(1):21–5.
57. American Thyroid Association (ATA) Guidelines Taskforce on Thyroid Nodules and Differentiated Thyroid Cancer, Cooper DS, Doherty GM, Haugen BR, et al. Revised American Thyroid Association management guidelines for patients with thyroid nodules and differentiated thyroid cancer. Thyroid 2009; 19(11):1167–214.
58. Jemal A, Siegel R, Ward E, et al. Cancer statistics, 2009. CA Cancer J Clin 2009; 59(4):225–49.
59. Dellal FD, Özdemir D, Tam AA, et al. Clinicopathological features of thyroid cancer in the elderly compared to younger counterparts: single-center experience. J Endocrinol Invest 2017;40(5):471–9.
60. van Tol KM, de Vries EG, Dullaart RP, et al. Differentiated thyroid carcinoma in the elderly. Crit Rev Oncol Hematol 2001;38(1):79–91.
61. Falvo L, Catania A, Sorrenti S, et al. Prognostic significance of the age factor in the thyroid cancer: statistical analysis. J Surg Oncol 2004;88(4):217–22.
62. Malloci A, Calo P, Nicolosi A, et al. Il carcinoma dellatiroide in eta geriatrica. Chirurgia (Bucur) 1998;11:6–8.
63. Rocco N, Amato B. Developing guidelines in geriatric surgery: role of the grade system. BMC Geriatr 2009;9(SUPPL 1):A99.
64. McConahey WM, Hay ID, Woolner LB, et al. Papillary thyroid cancer treated at the Mayo Clinic, 1946 through 1970: initial manifestations, pathologic findings, therapy, and outcome. Mayo Clin Proc 1986;61(12):978–96.
65. Ito Y, Kudo T, Kobayashi K, et al. Prognostic factors for recurrence of papillary thyroid carcinoma in the lymph nodes, lung, and bone: analysis of 5,768 patients with average 10-year follow-up. World J Surg 2012;36(6):1274–8.
66. Wu HS, Young MT, Ituarte PH, et al. Death from thyroid cancer of follicular cell origin. J Am Coll Surg 2000;191(6):600–6.
67. Davies L, Welch HG. Increasing incidence of thyroid cancer in the United States, 1973-2002. JAMA 2006;295(18):2164–7.
68. Castagna MG, Cantara S, Pacini F. Reappraisal of the indication for radioiodine thyroid ablation in differentiated thyroid cancer patients. J Endocrinol Invest 2016;39(10):1087–94.
69. Enewold L, Zhu K, Ron E, et al. Rising thyroid cancer incidence in the United States by demographic and tumor characteristics, 1980-2005. Cancer Epidemiol Biomarkers Prev 2009;18(3):784–91.
70. Mazzaferri EL, Jhiang SM. Long-term impact of initial surgical and medical therapy on papillary and follicular thyroid cancer. Am J Med 1994;97(5):418–28.
71. Kloos RT, Mazzaferri EL. A single recombinant human thyrotropin-stimulated serum thyroglobulin measurement predicts differentiated thyroid carcinoma metastases three to five years later. J Clin Endocrinol Metab 2005;90(9):5047–57.
72. Greene FL, Trotti A, Fritz AG, et al. Thyroid. In: Greene FL, Trotti A, Fritz AG, et al, editors. AJCC cancer staging handbook. 7th edition. Chicago: American Joint Committee on Cancer; 2010. p. 111–22.
73. Cady B, Rossi R. An expanded view of risk-group definition in differentiated thyroid carcinoma. Surgery 1988;104(6):947–53.

74. Mazzaferri E, Kloos R. Carcinoma of follicular epithelium: radioiodine and other treatments and outcomes. In: Braverman LE, Utiger RD, editors. Werner & Ingbar's the thyroid: a fundamental and clinical text, vol. 9. Philadelphia: Lippincott Williams Wilkins; 2005. p. 934–66.

75. SEER cancer statistics review (CSR). Surveillance, Epidemiology, and End Results program. 2013. Available at: http://seer.cancer.gov/csr/1975_2011. Accessed October 25, 2017.

76. Vini L, Hyer SL, Marshall J, et al. Long-term results in elderly patients with differentiated thyroid carcinoma. Cancer 2003;97(11):2736–42.

77. Park HS, Roman SA, Sosa JA. Treatment patterns of aging Americans with differentiated thyroid cancer. Cancer 2010;116(1):20–30.

78. Carcangiu ML, Zampi G, Pupi A, et al. Papillary carcinoma of the thyroid. A clinicopathologic study of 241 cases treated at the University of Florence, Italy. Cancer 1985;55(4):805–28.

79. Biliotti GC, Martini F, Vezzosi V, et al. Specific features of differentiated thyroid carcinoma in patients over 70 years of age. J Surg Oncol 2006;93(3):194–8.

80. Santangelo G, Del Giudice S, Gallucci F, et al. Cancer of the thyroid gland in geriatric age: a single center retrospective study with a 10-year postoperative follow-up. Int J Surg 2014;12(Suppl 2):S103–7.

81. Ito Y, Miyauchi A, Kihara M, et al. Patient age is significantly related to the progression of papillary microcarcinoma of the thyroid under observation. Thyroid 2014;24(1):27–34.

82. Sciuto R, Romano L, Rea S, et al. Natural history and clinical outcome of differentiated thyroid carcinoma: a retrospective analysis of 1503 patients treated at a single institution. Ann Oncol 2009;20(10):1728–35.

83. Neff RL, Farrar WB, Kloos RT, et al. Anaplastic thyroid cancer. Endocrinol Metab Clin North Am 2008;37(2):525–38, xi.

84. Takano T. Natural history of thyroid cancer [Review]. Endocr J 2017;64(3):237–44.

85. Toniato A, Boschin I, Casara D, et al. Papillary thyroid carcinoma: factors influencing recurrence and survival. Ann Surg Oncol 2008;15(5):1518–22.

86. Hung W, Sarlis NJ. Current controversies in the management of pediatric patients with well-differentiated nonmedullary thyroid cancer: a review. Thyroid 2002;12(8):683–702.

87. National Comprehensive Cancer Network (NCCN). NCCN clinical practice guidelines in oncology. 2012. Available at: https://www.nccn.org/professionals/physician_gls/f_guidelines_nojava.asp. Accessed October 25, 2017.

88. Jonklaas J, Sarlis NJ, Litofsky D, et al. Outcomes of patients with differentiated thyroid carcinoma following initial therapy. Thyroid 2006;16(12):1229–42.

89. McLeod DSA, Sawka AM, Cooper DS. Controversies in primary treatment of low-risk papillary thyroid cancer. Lancet 2013;381(9871):1046–57.

90. Xia Q, Dong S, Bian P-D, et al. Effects of endocrine therapy on the prognosis of elderly patients after surgery for papillary thyroid carcinoma. Eur Arch Otorhinolaryngol 2016;273(4):1037–43.

91. McLeod DSA, Carruthers K, Kevat DAS. Optimal differentiated thyroid cancer management in the elderly. Drugs Aging 2015;32(4):283–94.

92. Tuttle RM, Leboeuf R, Robbins RJ, et al. Empiric radioactive iodine dosing regimens frequently exceed maximum tolerated activity levels in elderly patients with thyroid cancer. J Nucl Med 2006;47(10):1587–91.

93. Ronga G, Filesi M, Montesano T, et al. Lung metastases from differentiated thyroid carcinoma. A 40 years' experience. Q J Nucl Med Mol Imaging 2004;48(1): 12–9.
94. Schlumberger M, Challeton C, De Vathaire F, et al. Radioactive iodine treatment and external radiotherapy for lung and bone metastases from thyroid carcinoma. J Nucl Med 1996;37(4):598–605.
95. Schwartz DL, Lobo MJ, Ang KK, et al. Postoperative external beam radiotherapy for differentiated thyroid cancer: outcomes and morbidity with conformal treatment. Int J Radiat Oncol Biol Phys 2009;74(4):1083–91.
96. Perros P, Boelaert K, Colley S, et al. Guidelines for the management of thyroid cancer. Clin Endocrinol (Oxf) 2014;81(Suppl 1):1–122.
97. Brose MS, Nutting CM, Jarzab B, et al. Sorafenib in radioactive iodine-refractory, locally advanced or metastatic differentiated thyroid cancer: a randomised, double-blind, phase 3 trial. Lancet 2014;384(9940):319–28.
98. Kapiteijn E, Schneider TC, Morreau H, et al. New treatment modalities in advanced thyroid cancer. Ann Oncol 2012;23(1):10–8.
99. Yun K-J, Kim W, Kim EH, et al. Accelerated disease progression after discontinuation of sorafenib in a patient with metastatic papillary thyroid cancer. Endocrinol Metab (Seoul) 2014;29(3):388–93.
100. Kim HJ, Sohn SY, Jang HW, et al. Multifocality, but not bilaterality, is a predictor of disease recurrence/persistence of papillary thyroid carcinoma. World J Surg 2013;37(2):376–84.
101. Miyauchi A, Kudo T, Kihara M, et al. Relationship of biochemically persistent disease and thyroglobulin-doubling time to age at surgery in patients with papillary thyroid carcinoma. Endocr J 2013;60(4):415–21.

Anesthesia in the Elderly Patient Undergoing Otolaryngology Head and Neck Surgery

Takumi Codère-Maruyama, MD, MSc*, Albert Moore, MD

KEYWORDS

- Anesthesia • Considerations • Geriatric • Otolaryngology • Surgery

KEY POINTS

- The proportion of geriatric patients presenting for surgery will continue to increase.
- The loss of functional reserve in the elderly has important clinical implications on the perioperative course.
- Mortality, morbidity, and the incidence of cognitive dysfunction is higher in the elderly, particularly in the frail patient.
- Preliminary evidence suggests that perioperative outcomes in the elderly can be improved with targeted interventions in the preoperative, intraoperative, and postoperative periods.

INTRODUCTION

The relationship between the otolaryngologist and anesthesiologist is unique among surgical specialties. Because of the proximity of the surgical site to the airway, otolaryngologic surgery requires collaboration between these 2 specialists and a mutual understanding of each other's practice. With the increasing number of elderly patients presenting for otolaryngologic surgery, appreciation of the impact of surgical and anesthetic treatments on the care of this special patient population is essential. In this review, an overview of the basic concepts and evolving challenges pertaining to the care of geriatric patients undergoing ear, note, and throat (ENT) procedures are presented from the perspective of the anesthesiologist.

Disclosure Statement: The authors have nothing to disclose.
Department of Anesthesia, McGill University Health Center, Glen site Royal Victoria Hospital, 1001 Boulevard Décarie, Room C05.2553, Montreal, Quebec H4A 3J1, Canada
* Corresponding author.
E-mail address: takumi.coderemaruyama@mcgill.ca

Clin Geriatr Med 34 (2018) 279–288
https://doi.org/10.1016/j.cger.2018.01.005
geriatric.theclinics.com

PHYSIOLOGY OF AGING

The primary concern for older patients is their progressive loss of functional reserve in all organ systems. This loss of reserve has implications in their daily lives and in the perioperative period. Even the healthy older adult has reduced physiologic reserve and is not spared from potential organ compromise during times of illness or surgical stress. The following physiologic changes should be considered when administering anesthetic care to the geriatric population.

Nervous System

Alterations in the central nervous and peripheral nervous system have an impact on the elderly patient's response to medications including anesthetics. Increased sensitivity to anesthetics can be observed after the age of 40.[1] The perception of pain also changes with age. Reduction in myelinated fibers and alterations at the nociceptors may account for higher pain thresholds observed in elderly.[2] Advancing age is accompanied by a gradual reduction of cerebral blood flow, reduction in brain size, and diminished production of neurotransmitters such as norepinephrine, dopamine, and acetylcholine.[3] With advancing age, the sympathetic outflow increases to compensate for the reduced cellular responsiveness to adrenergic stimulation. On the contrary, the parasympathetic activity decreases.[4] Clinically, decreases in brain reserve and changes in autonomic activity manifest as increased sensitivity to anesthetics, increased risks of perioperative delirium and cognitive dysfunction, compromised thermoregulation and hypothermia, and higher incidence of orthostatic hypotension and dehydration.

Cardiovascular System

Exertional capacity decreases with age. Progressive loss of vascular elasticity underlies the development of hypertension and left ventricular hypertrophy.[5] Vascular stiffening and autonomic changes commonly cause labile blood pressure with episodes of significant hypotension during anesthesia. As the ventricle hypertrophies, relaxation of the myocardium in diastole slows, and ventricular filling is impaired, a condition called *diastolic dysfunction*. Atrial contraction and elevated atrial pressure become important mediators of adequate diastolic filling. Episodes of atrial arrhythmias can easily cause hemodynamic instability, and fluid administration can result in pulmonary edema.[6] Although the presence and severity of diastolic dysfunction are commonly overlooked, most congestive heart failure in the elderly occurs in the absence of systolic dysfunction.[7] The incidence of coronary artery arteriosclerosis and valvular disease becomes higher with age and can further complicate the clinical picture.

Respiratory System

Increased chest wall stiffness and decreased lung parenchyma elasticity characterize the aging of the respiratory system.[8] A modest decline in resting partial pressure of oxygen and an increase in ventilation-perfusion mismatch further contributes to the decreased ability to compensate for a sudden increase in minute ventilation in the elderly.[9] The sensitivity of anesthetics in the geriatric age group puts them at risk for perioperative hypercarbia and hypoxemia. Furthermore, generalized loss of airway muscle tone with age predisposes older patients to aspiration pneumonitis and airway obstruction postoperatively.

Pharmacology

Pharmacokinetic and pharmacodynamic changes that accompany the aging process typically influence the sensitivity of the target organ to a given drug. A reduced total blood volume and a reduced protein binding contribute to a higher free concentration of medications, resulting in a more pronounced effect on older patients. Drug metabolism is also decreased because of a lower rate of clearance and a higher total volume of distribution.[10,11]

PERIOPERATIVE OUTCOMES IN THE ELDERLY PATIENTS
Mortality

Age, comorbidity, frailty and invasiveness of the surgical procedure are all predictors of mortality in geriatric patients.[12] Other studies have identified greatly advanced age ($\geq$85 years), emergency surgery, malnutrition, and the American Society of Anesthesiologists' ASA Physical Status classification system as additional risk factors for mortality and morbidity.[13–15] The risk of anesthesia-related mortality increases significantly in the oldest elderly patients ($\geq$85 years), with death rates of 20 per million as opposed to 8 per million in the general population.[16]

Morbidity

Cardiac and pulmonary complications
Although older adults have a higher prevalence of cardiovascular disease, age is not considered a major risk factor for major adverse cardiac events, according to the 2014 American College of Cardiology/American Heart Association perioperative guidelines.[17] On the contrary, an observational study has reported an increased incidence of perioperative adverse cardiovascular events in patients $\geq$68 years.[18]

The risk of perioperative pulmonary complications (atelectasis, pneumonia, respiratory failure, exacerbation of chronic lung disease) increases with increasing age.[19] Frailty and inadequate reversal of muscle relaxation after anesthesia can predispose to aspiration pneumonia and respiratory failure.[20]

Renal complications
Advanced age increases the risk of acute kidney injury. The adjusted hazard ratio for this adverse event is 1.7 in patients $\geq$56 years. However, when this occurs, the 30-day mortality rate is significantly augmented.[21]

Postoperative delirium and postoperative cognitive dysfunction
Postoperative delirium is reported to occur in up to 70% of patients $\geq$60 undergoing major surgery, and it is associated with higher mortality, permanent cognitive decline, and prolonged hospital stay.[22] Despite its high incidence, postoperative delirium remains poorly understood, and no one treatment can decrease its incidence or mitigate its duration. Important risk factors that have been identified to contribute to delirium include pain, dehydration, blood loss, metabolic imbalances, hypoxemia, and acute medical conditions. Certain drugs, such as anticholinergics, benzodiazepines, opioids, and steroids, have been described to precipitate delirium in vulnerable patients.[22] The use of the bispectral index to monitor and avoid unnecessarily deep anesthesia has been proposed as a technique to decrease delirium.[23]

Postoperative cognitive dysfunction (POCD) is a transient, or permanent, cognitive decline temporally associated with surgery and anesthesia. In fact, up to 50% of elderly patients undergoing surgery may be left with permanent cognitive decline.[24] Whether general anesthesia contributes to POCD remains unclear. This is illustrated by a meta-analysis comparing general versus regional anesthesia, which found no association between general anesthesia and development of POCD.[25] Hence, POCD is likely a manifestation of poor neurologic reserves unmasked by the perioperative stress.

ANESTHETIC STRATEGIES TO IMPROVE OUTCOME IN THE ELDERLY SURGICAL PATIENTS
Improved Assessment of the Elderly

Evaluation of reserve is an integral part of anesthetic assessment. The extreme diversity in health and functional independence of older individuals represents a challenge in the preoperative assessment. Although aging is associated with an inevitable decline in physiologic reserve, its extent varies from one individual to another, and the ability to cope with surgical stress and increased demand varies as well. Chronologic age itself is not an independent risk factor for perioperative cardiac morbidity and mortality. In fact, chronologic age and a list of comorbidities often fail to capture the patient's true physical condition or their capacity to withstand stress and inflammation associated with the procedure. The heterogeneity of the aging population confers additional challenges for clinicians to adequately risk stratify the geriatric patient. The term *frailty* has been increasingly used to describe a state of weakness, vulnerability, and a generalized decline in physiologic reserve and function, which exceeds what one would expect from advanced age alone.[26] The presence of frailty is a predictor of postoperative morbidity and mortality in emergency,[27] general,[28] orthopedic,[29] thoracic,[30] cardiac,[31] and even otolaryngologic surgery.[32] Indeed, frailty has a stronger association with morbidity or mortality than age or any distinct medical comorbidity.[33] Given the strong link between frailty and outcome, the ability to rapidly screen and accurately identify frail patients is important. Multiple methods of quantifying frailty have been validated.[34–39] Practical considerations have limited their utility in everyday clinical application. A universally accepted and standardized definition and measure of frailty is still lacking. Nevertheless, early recognition of the frail is important. Preliminary evidence suggests that the implementation of preoperative frailty screening and a special clinical pathway involving geriatric care principles can reduce 30-day mortality.[40]

Optimizing the Geriatric Patient

A reduction in cardiorespiratory reserves puts the geriatric patient at risk of being unable to tolerate the increased oxygen requirements after surgery. The resulting oxygen debt puts strain on the various organ systems, increasing the risk of organ failure and complications. This can have real consequences in the elderly, as those with lower anaerobic thresholds are found to have increased mortality and those with lower walking capacity have worse postoperative outcome.[41,42] The idea of prehabilitation, in which the elderly patient is physically and nutritionally optimized before surgery to modulate perioperative outcome, has evolved into a hot research and clinical topic in the last decade.[43] Prehabilitation typically uses a multimodal intervention involving aerobic and resistance training, psychological care, and nutritional supplementation about 4 weeks before surgery. Small recent randomized, controlled trials found that such prehabilitation regimens led to earlier recovery of the patients' functional capacity, as assessed with the 6-minute walk test, and have better postoperative recovery when compared with rehabilitation or standard care.[44,45] Although most of the literature investigating the effects of prehabilitation have involved colorectal surgery, these concepts are presumably applicable to any geriatric patient undergoing any type of surgery. Nevertheless, such an extensive prehabilitation regimen may be exaggerated for a short, less-invasive procedure. Nutritional supplementation alone may possibly confer a certain cost-effective benefit in specific geriatric subpopulations by decreasing postoperative complication rates.[46] Additional research and efforts are needed to develop a methodic approach to identify frailty and devise individualized prehabilitation regimens relative to the intended procedure.

Inhalation Versus Total Intravenous Anesthesia

Total intravenous anesthesia (TIVA) is achieved with a continuous infusion of propofol together with an opioid. This anesthetic strategy is commonly used in airway surgery, when administration of inhalational agents is precluded by the use of jet ventilation. Remifentanil is an ultra–short-acting opioid agonist which is ideal for highly stimulating head and neck surgeries. The brevity of action of this drug and the noncumulative effects even after a prolonged infusion time, make it ideal for highly stimulating procedures of any duration, such as laryngoscopies. Hemodynamic fluctuations owing to alternating intervals of high and minimal surgical stimulation can also be attenuated by remifentanil. Bucking and bleeding from the surgical site at emergence can be minimized, owing to the predictable elimination pattern of this opioid. Multiple trials have evaluated TIVA as a mean to decrease vasodilation and blood loss while improving surgical view.[47–49] Although some studies found significant improvement in surgical field, others did not. A Cochrane review on this matter concluded that TIVA does not decrease total blood loss yet may slightly improve the quality of the surgical field.[50]

Improved Muscle Relaxation Strategy

Intraoperative muscle relaxation is an essential component of endoscopic and laryngeal surgeries. The administration of intermediate-duration nondepolarizing neuromuscular blocking agents provides profound degrees of muscle relaxation that contributes significantly to optimal surgical views and conditions. However, from the anesthesiologist's point of view, the profound block often needed until the very end of the surgery can be difficult to reverse and may delay return of airway reflexes and extubation. Postoperative residual muscle relaxation has been reported to occur in 40% of patients after admission to the postanesthesia care unit.[51] The risk of residual blockade is increased in laryngeal surgery, in which most procedures take less than 30 minutes. This is particularly true in older patients, whose age-related reductions in hepatic and renal excretion can prolong the duration of action of some commonly used neuromuscular blocking agents (eg, rocuronium). Even small amounts of residual neuromuscular block can impair pharyngeal and swallowing functions, predisposing the elderly patient to aspiration pneumonia.[20] The introduction of sugammadex, a selective relaxant-binding agent, may resolve this conflict between optimal surgical conditions and anesthetic implications. Sugammadex can rapidly achieve reversal of neuromuscular block by binding to rocuronium molecules, thereby preventing them from functioning at the neuromuscular junction. Dose-finding studies have found that sugammadex was effective in reversing rocuronium-induced muscle relaxation, including profound blockade.[52,53] Kim and colleagues[54] prospectively assessed the effect of deep versus moderate neuromuscular blockade on surgical conditions during laryngeal microsurgery, using sugammadex to reverse deep neuromuscular blockade. The surgeon involved in this study reported a lower resistance to rigid laryngoscopy and an easier exposure of the vocal cords in patients allocated to receive deep neuromuscular blockade. The incidence of vocal cord movements during surgery was also reported to be significantly lower in this group. The authors conclude that the use of deep neuromuscular blockade, reversed with sugammadex at the end of surgery, significantly improved surgical conditions during laryngeal microsurgery. However, the study was unblinded, and more data are needed to confirm these findings. Of note, although sugammadex is found to be well tolerated by patients of all ages, elderly patients take a slightly longer time to recover muscle function after the administration of sugammadex.[55]

Monitored Anesthesia Care

Monitored anesthesia care (MAC) has gained attention as a safe way to provide sedation and analgesia, especially among elderly patients requiring a diagnostic or therapeutic procedure. This anesthetic strategy has the advantage of avoiding general anesthesia in a frail or medically compromised patient, and hence is considered a first anesthetic choice in selected surgical procedures. During the MAC technique, the goal of the anesthesiologist is to administer a combination of short-acting medications to provide sedation, anxiolysis, and analgesia while maintaining spontaneous respiration and airway reflexes. This technique also helps hasten the recovery after the procedure. An ideal sedative agent should have a rapid onset, a high clearance, and minimal side effects and be easily titratable. Because older patients are more sensitive to the effects of anesthetics, the administration of drugs should be incremental, and the clinician should remain vigilant on the possibility of airway obstruction, hypoxemia, hypercarbia, or aspiration. The standard of care for patients undergoing MAC is the same for patients undergoing general anesthesia and does not preclude the need for a thorough preoperative assessment, standard monitoring, and postanesthesia care.[56] Although there are various medications (eg ketamine, propofol, midazolam) to achieve the desired sedation and analgesia, the newer drug dexmedetomidine has gained particular attention in the last decades. Dexmedetomidine, a selective and potent α-2 adrenergic receptor agonist, acts on the sleep pathway and causes minimal respiratory depression, contrary to drugs that act on γ-aminobutyric acid (GABA) receptors (eg midazolam, propofol). Its sympatholytic action attenuates blood pressure and heart rate responses to surgical stimulation.[57] The result is a calm and sedated patient who can easily be aroused. The routine use of dexmedetomidine may however be limited by its half-life of 2 to 3 hours. The development of severe bradycardia, hypotension, and even cardiac arrest can also limit its clinical usefulness.[58] The use of an α-2 receptor agonist such as clonidine or dexmedetomidine may be of particular interest in certain ENT surgeries, especially when spontaneous ventilation needs to be preserved until a definitive airway can be secured. Few studies have evaluated the efficacy of these drugs as an adjuvant in anesthesia for ENT surgeries. Kumari and colleagues[59] reported a safe and effective use of intravenous clonidine as an adjuvant to MAC in elective ENT surgeries. The patients who received a continuous intraoperative infusion of clonidine required less rescue sedative and analgesic and had lower heart rates and blood pressures, less bleeding in the surgical field, and higher surgeon and patient satisfaction. Other reports have described dexmedetomidine as an effective primary agent for MAC in neurosurgical, ophthalmologic, and ENT procedures in adult patients.[60–62] However, the occurrence of cardiovascular depression and delayed recovery room discharge have been raised as concerns when choosing this drug.[61] Another benefit of dexmedetomidine is its potential ability to reduce the incidence and duration of postoperative delirium in the elderly.[63–66] Dexmedetomidine may have an intrinsic protective effect on delirium, beyond the simple avoidance of GABA agonists.[66] Yet these findings are mostly from trials performed in the intensive care unit and do not necessarily prompt the use of prophylactic dexmedetomidine for the prevention of delirium in all geriatric postoperative patients. Finally, a recently published study has investigated the use of oral pregabalin as another adjuvant for MAC during ENT surgery. The oral administration of pregabalin, 150 mg 1 hour before surgery, led to not only a decrease in intraoperative propofol and fentanyl requirements but also lesser requirements of analgesics in the postoperative period.[67] A perfect MAC recipe that fits all patient is unlikely to exist. Nevertheless, additional investigations and use of these drugs could confer significant benefits to physiologically and metabolically handicapped elderly adults by lowering surgical stress, pain, and incidence of delirium and hastening recovery from anesthesia.

SUMMARY

Geriatric patients undergoing surgery have a whole set of specific physiologic changes, perioperative needs, and postoperative complications. Clinically, elderly patients are distinct from their younger adult counterparts, and hence require specialized and individualized treatment pathways. Decrease in physiologic reserves, altered pharmacokinetics and pharmacodynamics, frailty, postoperative delirium, and cognitive decline are all issues specific to the elderly that can significantly impact the outcome. Yet, we are only starting to understand the mechanisms of these conditions, and more research is needed as to how we can improve geriatric perioperative care from preoperative assessment to the provision of targeted interventions. With the aging of the baby boomers, combined with significant medical advances that allow people to live longer than ever, otolaryngologists and anesthesiologists will likely have to face an increasing number of medically and surgically challenging cases in this patient population. As perioperative physicians, we need to increase our awareness and understanding of the multitude of problems associated with the geriatric patient undergoing surgery.

REFERENCES

1. Mapleson W. Effect of age on MAC in humans: a meta-analysis. Br J Anaesth 1996;76(2):179–85.
2. Gibson SJ, Farrell M. A review of age differences in the neurophysiology of nociception and the perceptual experience of pain. Clin J pain 2004;20(4):227–39.
3. Peters R. Ageing and the brain. Postgrad Med J 2006;82(964):84–8.
4. Collins KJ. The autonomic nervous system in old age. Rev Clin Gerontol 1991; 1(4):337–45.
5. Barodka VM, Joshi BL, Berkowitz DE, et al. Implications of vascular aging. Anesth Analg 2011;112(5):1048–60.
6. Groban L, Butterworth J. Perioperative management of chronic heart failure. Anesth Analg 2006;103(3):557–75.
7. Lakatta EG. Cardiovascular aging in health. Clin Geriatr Med 2000;16(3):419–43.
8. Janssens JP, Pache JC, Nicod LP. Physiological changes in respiratory function associated with ageing. Eur Respir J 1999;13(1):197–205.
9. Zaugg M, Lucchinetti E. Respiratory function in the elderly. Anesthesiol Clin North America 2000;18(1):47–58.
10. Esposito C, Plati A, Mazzullo T, et al. Renal function and functional reserve in healthy elderly individuals. J Nephrol 2007;20(5):617–25.
11. Rivera R, Antognini JF. Perioperative drug therapy in elderly patients. Anesthesiology 2009;110(5):1176–81.
12. Hamel MB, Henderson WG, Khuri SF, et al. Surgical outcomes for patients aged 80 and older: morbidity and mortality from major noncardiac surgery. J Am Geriatr Soc 2005;53(3):424–9.
13. Pelavski AD, De Miguel M, Garcia-Tejedor GA, et al. Mortality, geriatric, and nongeriatric surgical risk factors among the eldest old: a prospective observational study. Anesth Analg 2017;125(4):1329–36.

14. Hosking MP, Warner MA, Lobdell CM, et al. Outcomes of surgery in patients 90 years of age and older. Jama 1989;261(13):1909–15.
15. van Diepen S, Bakal JA, McAlister FA, et al. Mortality and readmission of patients with heart failure, atrial fibrillation, or coronary artery disease undergoing noncardiac surgery. Circulation 2011;124(3):289–96.
16. Li G, Warner M, Lang BH, et al. Epidemiology of anesthesia-related mortality in the United States, 1999–2005. Anesthesiology 2009;110(4):759–65.
17. Fleisher LA, Fleischmann KE, Auerbach AD, et al. 2014 ACC/AHA guideline on perioperative cardiovascular evaluation and management of patients undergoing noncardiac surgery. Circulation 2014;130:e278–333.
18. Kheterpal S, O'Reilly M, Englesbe MJ, et al. Preoperative and intraoperative predictors of cardiac adverse events after general, vascular, and urological surgery. Anesthesiology 2009;110(1):58–66.
19. Smetana GW, Lawrence VA, Cornell JE. Preoperative pulmonary risk stratification for noncardiothoracic surgery: systematic review for the american college of physicianspreoperative pulmonary risk stratification for noncardiothoracic surgery. Ann Intern Med 2006;144(8):581–95.
20. Cedborg AIH, Sundman E, Bodén K, et al. Pharyngeal function and breathing pattern during partial neuromuscular block in the elderlyeffects on airway protection. Anesthesiology 2014;120(2):312–25.
21. Kheterpal S, Tremper KK, Heung M, et al. Development and validation of an acute kidney injury risk index for patients undergoing general surgeryresults from a national data set. Anesthesiology 2009;110(3):505–15.
22. Schenning KJ, Deiner SG. Postoperative delirium: a review of risk factors and tools of prediction. Curr Anesthesiol Rep 2015;5(1):48–56.
23. Chan MT, Cheng BC, Lee TM, et al. BIS-guided anesthesia decreases postoperative delirium and cognitive decline. J Neurosurg Anesthesiol 2013;25(1):33–42.
24. McDonagh DL, Mathew JP, White WD, et al. Cognitive function after major noncardiac surgery, apolipoprotein E4 genotype, and biomarkers of brain injury. Anesthesiology 2010;112(4):852–9.
25. Guay J. General anaesthesia does not contribute to long-term post-operative cognitive dysfunction in adults: a meta-analysis. Indian J Anaesth 2011;55(4):358–63.
26. Clegg A, Young J, Iliffe S, et al. Frailty in elderly people. Lancet 2013;381(9868):752–62.
27. Du Y, Karvellas CJ, Baracos V, et al. Sarcopenia is a predictor of outcomes in very elderly patients undergoing emergency surgery. Surgery 2014;156(3):521–7.
28. Lasithiotakis K, Petrakis J, Venianaki M, et al. Frailty predicts outcome of elective laparoscopic cholecystectomy in geriatric patients. Surg Endosc 2013;27(4):1144–50.
29. Patel KV, Brennan KL, Brennan ML, et al. Association of a modified frailty index with mortality after femoral neck fracture in patients aged 60 years and older. Clin Orthop Relat Res 2014;472(3):1010–7.
30. Tsiouris A, Hammoud ZT, Velanovich V, et al. A modified frailty index to assess morbidity and mortality after lobectomy. J Surg Res 2013;183(1):40–6.
31. Bagnall NM, Faiz O, Darzi A, et al. What is the utility of preoperative frailty assessment for risk stratification in cardiac surgery? Interact Cardiovasc Thorac Surg 2013;17(2):398–402.
32. Adams P, Ghanem T, Stachler R, et al. Frailty as a predictor of morbidity and mortality in inpatient head and neck surgery. JAMA Otolaryngol Head Neck Surg 2013;139(8):783–9.

33. Winograd CH, Gerety MB, Chung M, et al. Screening for frailty: criteria and predictors of outcomes. J Am Geriatr Soc 1991;39(8):778–84.
34. Fried LP, Tangen CM, Walston J, et al. Frailty in older adults: evidence for a phenotype. J Gerontol A Biol Sci Med Sci 2001;56(3):M146–57.
35. Mitnitski AB, Mogilner AJ, Rockwood K. Accumulation of deficits as a proxy measure of aging. ScientificWorldJournal 2001;1:323–36.
36. Velanovich V, Antoine H, Swartz A, et al. Accumulating deficits model of frailty and postoperative mortality and morbidity: its application to a national database. J Surg Res 2013;183(1):104–10.
37. George EM, Burke WM, Hou JY, et al. Measurement and validation of frailty as a predictor of outcomes in women undergoing major gynaecological surgery. BJOG 2016;123(3):455–61.
38. Shin JI, Keswani A, Lovy AJ, et al. Simplified frailty index as a predictor of adverse outcomes in total hip and knee arthroplasty. J Arthroplasty 2016; 31(11):2389–94.
39. Saliba D, Elliott M, Rubenstein LZ, et al. The vulnerable elders survey: a tool for identifying vulnerable older people in the community. J Am Geriatr Soc 2001; 49(12):1691–9.
40. Hall DE, Arya S, Schmid KK, et al. Association of a frailty screening initiative with postoperative survival at 30, 180, and 365 days. JAMA Surg 2017;152(3):233–40.
41. Older R, Smith R, Courtney B, et al. Preoperative evaluation of cardiac failure and ischemia in elderly patients by cardiopulmonary exercise testing. Chest 1993; 104(3):701–4.
42. Lee L, Schwartzman K, Carli F, et al. The association of the distance walked in 6 min with pre-operative peak oxygen consumption and complications 1 month after colorectal resection. Anaesthesia 2013;68(8):811–6.
43. Hulzebos E, van Meeteren N. Making the elderly fit for surgery. Br J Surg 2016; 103(2):e12–5.
44. Li C, Carli F, Lee L, et al. Impact of a trimodal prehabilitation program on functional recovery after colorectal cancer surgery: a pilot study. Surg Endosc 2013;27(4):1072–82.
45. Gillis C, Li C, Lee L, et al. Prehabilitation versus REHABILITATIONA randomized control trial in patients undergoing colorectal resection for cancer. Anesthesiology 2014;121(5):937–47.
46. Liu M, Yang J, Yu X, et al. The role of perioperative oral nutritional supplementation in elderly patients after hip surgery. Clin Interv Aging 2015;10:849–58.
47. Ahn H, Chung SK, Dhong HJ, et al. Comparison of surgical conditions during propofol or sevoflurane anaesthesia for endoscopic sinus surgery. Br J Anaesth 2007;100(1):50–4.
48. Eberhart LH, Folz BJ, Wulf H, et al. Intravenous anesthesia provides optimal surgical conditions during microscopic and endoscopic sinus surgery. Laryngoscope 2003;113(8):1369–73.
49. Beule AG, Wilhelmi F, Kühnel TS, et al. Propofol versus sevoflurane: bleeding in endoscopic sinus surgery. Otolaryngol Head Neck Surg 2007;136(1):45–50.
50. Boonmak S, Boonmak P, Laopaiboon M. Deliberate hypotension with propofol under anaesthesia for functional endoscopic sinus surgery (FESS). Cochrane Database Syst Rev 2013;(6):CD006623.
51. Murphy GS, Brull SJ. Residual neuromuscular block: lessons unlearned. Part I: definitions, incidence, and adverse physiologic effects of residual neuromuscular block. Anesth Analgesia 2010;111(1):120–8.

52. Pühringer FK, Rex C, Sielenkämper AW, et al. Reversal of profound, high-dose rocuronium–induced meeting abstracts by sugammadex at two different time pointsan international, multicenter, randomized, dose-finding, safety assessor-blinded, phase II trial. Anesthesiology 2008;109(2):188–97.
53. Suy K, Morias K, Cammu G, et al. Effective reversal of moderate rocuronium-or vecuronium-induced neuromuscular block with sugammadex, a selective relaxant binding agent. Anesthesiology 2007;106(2):283–8.
54. Kim H, Lee K, Park W, et al. Deep neuromuscular block improves the surgical conditions for laryngeal microsurgery. Br J Anaesth 2015;115(6):867–72.
55. McDonagh DL, Benedict PE, Kovac AL, et al. Efficacy, safety, and pharmacokinetics of sugammadex for the reversal of rocuronium-induced meeting abstracts in elderly patients. Anesthesiology 2011;114(2):318–29.
56. American Society of Anesthesiologists. Position on monitored anesthesia care. Last amended October 16, 2013.
57. Kamibayashi T, Maze M. Clinical uses of α2-adrenergic agonists. Anesthesiology 2000;93(5):1345–9.
58. Ingersoll-Weng E, Manecke GR, Thistlethwaite PA. Dexmedetomidine and cardiac arrest. Anesthesiology 2004;100(3):738–9.
59. Kumari I, Naithani U, Singhal Y, et al. Clonidine as an adjuvant in monitored anesthesia care for ENT surgeries: a prospective, randomized, double blind placebo controlled study. Anaesth Pain Intensive Care 2015;19(3):260–8.
60. Bishnoi V, Kumar B, Bhagat H, et al. Comparison of dexmedetomidine versus midazolam-fentanyl combination for monitored anesthesia care during burr-hole surgery for chronic subdural hematoma. J Neurosurg anesthesiology 2016; 28(2):141–6.
61. Alhashemi J. Dexmedetomidine vs midazolam for monitored anaesthesia care during cataract surgery. BJA: Br J Anaesth 2006;96(6):722–6.
62. Busick T, Kussman M, Scheidt T, et al. Preliminary experience with dexmedetomidine for monitored anesthesia care during ENT surgical procedures. Am J Ther 2008;15(6):520–7.
63. Riker RR, Shehabi Y, Bokesch PM, et al. Dexmedetomidine vs midazolam for sedation of critically ill patients: a randomized trial. Jama 2009;301(5):489–99.
64. Pandharipande PP, Pun BT, Herr DL, et al. Effect of sedation with dexmedetomidine vs lorazepam on acute brain dysfunction in mechanically ventilated patients: the MENDS randomized controlled trial. Jama 2007;298(22):2644–53.
65. Djaiani G, Silverton N, Fedorko L, et al. Dexmedetomidine versus propofol sedation reduces delirium after cardiac surgery: a randomized controlled trial. Anesthesiology 2016;124(2):362–8.
66. Su X, Meng ZT, Wu XH, et al. Dexmedetomidine for prevention of delirium in elderly patients after non-cardiac surgery: a randomised, double-blind, placebo-controlled trial. Lancet 2016;388(10054):1893–902.
67. Kochhar A, Banday J, Ahmad Z, et al. Pregabalin in monitored anesthesia care for ear-nose-throat surgery. Anesth Essays Res 2017;11(2):350–3.

Frailty and Polypharmacy in Older Patients with Otolaryngologic Diseases

David Eibling, MD

KEYWORDS

- Frailty • Polypharmacy • Balance disorders in the elderly • Dysphagia in the elderly
- Surgical decision making in the elderly
- National Surgical Quality Improvement Project
- Veterans Administration Surgical Quality Improvement Project
- Risk assessment index

KEY POINTS

- Within the specialty of otolaryngology, frailty is primarily manifested in older adults through increased risk for falls, dysfunctional swallowing, and impairment of pulmonary function delaying recovery after surgery.
- Multiple measures of frailty exist, some of which are tailored to assist in surgical decision making.
- Although knowledge of frailty and its implications is gradually increasing among otolaryngologists, dramatic knowledge gaps exist that impair care for older patients.
- Polypharmacy leads to considerable morbidity among older patients with otolaryngologic diseases, particularly those with balance disorders, xerostomia, and dysphagia.

INTRODUCTION

Numerous disorders commonly managed by otolaryngologists, specialists in diseases of the ear, nose, and sinuses; upper aerodigestive tract; and neck, are affected by aging. Several of these disorders are significantly impacted by frailty and overmedication. The readership of the *Geriatric Clinics of North America* is well aware of the science and clinical impact of frailty and overmedication and many of the specific comorbidities precipitated by frailty and overmedication. Unfortunately, clinical practice suggests this knowledge eludes most nongeriatric providers, including many otolaryngologists. This article reviews the salient points of how frailty impacts older patients with otolaryngologic disorders and the often unappreciated role of

The author has nothing to disclose.
Department of Otolaryngology–Head and Neck Surgery, VA Pittsburgh Healthcare System, University Drive C, Pittsburgh, PA 15240, USA
E-mail address: eiblingde@upmc.edu

Clin Geriatr Med 34 (2018) 289–298
https://doi.org/10.1016/j.cger.2018.01.006
geriatric.theclinics.com

overmedication. The reader is encouraged to use this information, and other knowledge, in education of nongeriatricians.

FRAILTY

Frailty as a syndrome, and the science underlying it, is well known to the readership of this issue of the *Clinics*. Consequently, this introduction will be abbreviated. A designation of "frail" implies a lack of sufficient physiologic reserve to withstand stressors and is associated with an increased likelihood of death within 5 years. Frailty is independent of age or a specific disease process and cannot be assessed by a single test or laboratory value. It represents a compilation of multiple processes, including sarcopenia or progressive loss of muscle tissue. Together, these processes result in reduced physiologic reserve. Although the term *frail* is commonly applied to descriptions of older adults, when used in the context of health care delivery, it conveys more specific meaning and has broad implications for patients and their care givers.

SPECIFIC IMPLICATIONS FOR FRAILTY IN OTOLARYNGOLOGY

The 3 areas in which frailty most commonly affects otolaryngologic disease processes are balance, swallowing, and surgical outcomes. All of these are substantially impacted by alterations in neuromuscular function and numerous other systems. Adequate core muscle strength is required for balance as is neural function to support proprioceptive and vestibular contributions. Adequate tongue, oral, glottic, and pharyngeal strength is required for effective swallowing, which means adequate swallowing without aspiration. Substantial data link tongue strength and glottic closure strength to swallowing function. These disorders and the role of weakness in their development are discussed in more detail in the article by Leila J. Mady and colleagues, "Head and Neck Cancer in the Elderly: Frailty, Shared Decisions, and Avoidance of Low Value Care", in this issue. Both disorders of balance and swallowing are also heavily impacted by polypharmacy, which are addressed in the closing paragraphs of this article.

FRAILTY AND SURGICAL OUTCOMES

Without question, the area in which frailty has been most actively investigated by surgical investigators is in the postoperative course of older adults after surgical procedures. Surgery is inherently stressful and has been likened to "running a 5K." Surgical procedures involving the upper airway, those requiring general anesthesia, and procedures affecting respiration or deglutition have the potential to "tip" the frail weak older individual into respiratory failure and a host of other disorders such as postoperative delirium. Aspiration (saliva or feedings) is common after seemingly unrelated upper airway surgery. Those with adequate reserve (near the fit end of the continuum) are able to accommodate by increased respiratory effort, cough, and early ambulation with increased pulmonary excursion. However, those who are frail—often bed ridden, weak, frequently with poor laryngo-pharyngeal function—may not recover adequate function after the stress of surgery. This situation may lead to prolonged hospitalization and even reintubation, postoperative pneumonia, and the requirement for long-term care in skilled nursing facilities. Several studies identified the implications both in terms of mortality and in the risk for complications.

Makary and coauthors[1] at Johns Hopkins used a modification of the Cardiovascular Health Study (CHS), a physical phenotype to be described later, to prospectively assess nearly 600 patients older than 65 undergoing elective surgery. Patients that scored 4 to 5 on a 5-point scale were considered frail. Frailty (independently) predicted increased risk of complications, prolonged hospitalization, and discharge to either a skilled nursing facility or an assisted living facility. Notably, their study found that the addition of a frailty measure improved the reliability of common preoperative risk assessment measures such as the American Society of Anesthesiologists score. Adams and colleagues[2] from Wayne State University used the modified frailty index (mFI) (primarily medical comorbidities (**Box 1**)) and risk assessment data in the American College of Surgeons National Surgical Quality Improvement Project (ACS–NSQIP) to evaluate the impact of frailty on inpatient head and neck surgical patients. Their cohort included data on 6727 patients undergoing common inpatient procedures, including thyroid, salivary, pharynx and tonsil, and neck dissection. One-half had mFI scores of 0, and fewer than 5% had scores higher than 0.27. Nevertheless, increasing mFI scores correlated closely with risk of grade 4 complications on the Clavien-Dindo scale, prolonged hospitalization, and 30-day mortality rate. Revenig and coauthors[3] at Emory University used a composite of the Hopkins frailty index to prospectively assess risk in a cohort of 189 patients undergoing elective surgery. They noted the phenotype score combined with the hemoglobin most accurately predicted wound complications, again using the Clavien-Dindo scale. Recently, Selb and coauthors[4] used the mFI to evaluate frailty in a cohort of 140,828 patients older than 40 undergoing ambulatory surgery accrued into the NSQIP database over a 4-year period from 2007 through 2010. Common procedures included thyroid/parathyroid, breast, and hernia. Despite the fact that no inpatients were included, the surgical complexity was similar to that of the Adams inpatient study. Less than 1% of the cohort studied experienced severe complications; however, the mFI correlated closely with the risk of complications. Those with a mFI greater than 0.36 had nearly a 4-fold risk for serious complications.

CHALLENGES OF FRAILTY ASSESSMENT IN CLINICAL SETTINGS

Identification of at-risk individuals should, therefore, represent "low-hanging fruit." Not only must at-risk frail patients be identified, but some sort of intervention to assist in either optimizing the patient for surgery or selection of alternative management strategy has the potential to reduce what Mady and colleagues term *low value care* in their article in this issue of *the Clinics*.

Box 1
Modified frailty index

Functional Status 2 or greater
  History of:
    Diabetes mellitus
    Chronic obstructive pulmonary disease or pneumonia
    Congestive heart failure
    Myocardial infarction
    Prior coronary stenting, angina
    Hypertension requiring medication
    Peripheral vascular disease or rest pain
    Impaired sensorium
    Transient ischemic attack or cerebrovascular accident
    Cerebrovascular accident with neurologic sequelae

Data from Adams P, Ghanem T, Stachler R, et al. Frailty as a predictor of morbidity and mortality in inpatient head and neck surgery. JAMA Otolaryngol Head Neck Surg 2013;138:783–9.

Outpatient otolaryngologic care is typically episodic, and not longitudinal, as is the usual situation in primary care practices. Moreover, with few exceptions, otolaryngology practices tend to be high throughput, with little time for solicitation of history that is (seemingly) unrelated to the chief complaint. Otolaryngologists, as a specialty, have difficulty managing patients with multiple comorbidities, often relying on their patient's primary care practitioners to identify, prioritize, and manage comorbidities such as anticoagulation and diabetes. As a result of this practice style, otolaryngologists may not recognize the stage of decline represented by a frail patient when encountered in a single visit. Vague comments from family members such as "she is slipping" may not be recognized as an indication of increasing frailty, potentially leading to inappropriate care decisions. Because the degree of decline may contribute substantially to the ongoing disease process for which the patient sought care and, even more dramatically, to the outcome of the intervention, recognition of frailty becomes critical. As others have noted, the challenge of the practitioner is to accurately position the patient on the continuum between frail and fit with the goal of optimizing preoperative decision making.

MEASURES OF FRAILTY

The overarching goal of quantifying frailty would be to identify at-risk patients before the condition becomes obvious. Because frailty represents loss of reserve in multiple homeostatic systems, measures draw from a wide range of indices, not a single system. Ideally, a single reliable measure of frailty would be widely used to identify where the patient lies between the extremes of frail and fit. Unfortunately, such a measure does not exist, for reasons that are discussed later in this section. As a result, communication among members of multidisciplinary care teams regarding the degree of frailty for a specific patient is often ineffectual. Even when aware of frailty measures, team members may use specific measures and be unaware of how they relate to those used by team members of other disciplines.

A recent publication by Dent and coauthors[5] reviewed 422 published articles and identified 29 different frailty measures. They observed that although creation of a single standardized assessment tool would seem to be a desirable goal for the geriatric community, such a tool is unlikely to be forthcoming because of the variability in goals and setting. The reader is referred to this heavily referenced review (127 references).

Among the most important reasons leading to the existence of multiple disparate measures is that there is no single definition of frailty; therefore, different measures were developed for specific, and disparate, purposes. Measures intended to predict the risk of frailty-induced falls likely require different elements than those that might predict postoperative recovery after cardiac surgery. Moreover, ease of data collection inevitably impacts the actual utility of the assessment. Comprehensive evaluations such as the Minimum Data Set (MDS) or the Comprehensive Geriatric Assessment serve a valuable role in establishing highly concise measures that can heavily influence treatment decisions, but are often not practical for use in routine clinical settings. The advent of computerized information systems has impacted data collection, but the extent of and accuracy of data entered and the ability to extract useful information is still imperfect. Until recently, data extraction has been limited to structured data; either ordinal, templated, or abstracted from text such as is used by standardized surgical databases, which is addressed later in this section. Data needed for research or for validation of preliminary screening assessment tools must necessarily be more detailed and include discrete outcomes data to assure high reliability.

CARDIOVASCULAR HEALTH STUDY ASSESSMENT TOOL

The most commonly used phenotype assessment is derived from the CHS tool, which is similar to the Frieds Frailty Phenotype, and can be found on the American Geriatric Society (AGS) website[6]: (http://geriatricscareonline.org/SearchResult/index/index/category_name/Frailty accessed 20 October 2017). Because it is likely the measure most familiar to the readers of this issue of *The Clinics*, it is not reproduced here. The CHS measure requires a brief history and observation of the patient to assess the extent or degree of involvement of 5 factors: (1) *shrinking* (unintentional weight loss), (2) weakness (low grip strength), (3) *exhaustion* (self-reported), (4) slowness (walking speed), and (5) low physical activity. A useful data collection tool can be found on the AGS Web site. Modifications of this assessment may be referred to by other terms, such as the *Hopkins Frailty Score* as in the review by Revenig and colleagues.[3]

MEASURES OF FRAILTY USED IN SURGICAL OUTCOMES STUDIES

It is safe to say that most surgeons (and most otolaryngologists) who treat older patients recognize the significance of frailty but are unfamiliar with the CHS. Frailty measures in the surgical literature differ substantially from those in the geriatric literature and often contain elements obtainable from review of the patient's chart or from large surgical risk assessment databases. These measures may blur the line between classic descriptions of frailty and generic comorbidities, presenting challenges to interpretation of published reports.

MODIFIED FRAILTY INDEX

The mFI has been used in several studies cited in this article and is described in detail by Adams and colleagues.[2] The mFI was derived from the 70-element Canadian Study of Health and Aging Frailty Index (CSHA-FI). Investigators mapped 11 variables from the CSHA-FI to variables present in the NSQIP database. These variables are listed in **Box 1** and are essentially medical comorbidities, data that can be easily extracted from chart review. Despite the fact that the mFI includes no phenotype assessment, studies such as those reviewed above find that these measures reliably predict frailty-related surgical outcomes. The mFI is presented as a decimal, in which 0 is no frailty, and a score greater than 0.44 represents severe frailty.

RISK ANALYSIS INDEX

The Risk Analysis Index (RAI) was developed within the Veteran's Administration (VA) with the goal of creating a clinical measure of frailty that could be easily administered, facilitating its use in a clinical setting to assist with decision making regarding elective surgery. It was described as a 2-part measure, a prospective clinical assessment based on patient questionnaire (RAI-C) and an administrative assessment (RAI-A) to be used for retrospective analysis and measure validation.[7] Current updates are being developed with different numeric scores, and the reader is encouraged to search for updated versions that may have been published by the time this issue of *The Clinics* has been released.

The RAI-C was derived from elements of the MDS Mortality Risk Index-Revised, with the goal of developing a reliable frailty measure that was easy to administer and that could identify frail patients before they arrive in the operating room. The initial validation cohort included 6856 unique VA patients, the report of which was published in *JAMA Surgery* in February 2017. The elements of the RAI-C are obtained by questioning the patient or caregiver and can be easily completed during routine nursing intake interview in about 2 minutes. The elements as published in 2017 are shown in **Box 2**. The score for age is modified by the presence of malignancy so that a diagnosis of metastatic or advanced cancer adds a variable number of points to the score. Male gender automatically adds 5 points. Scores for Activities of Daily Living (ADL) are heavily impacted by the presence of cognitive decline. A total score of 21 or greater is interpreted as frail (in the 2017 version). Newer versions under development will have different schemata and different cutoff points. The RAI-C is now in active clinical use at the author's institutions, both within the University of Pittsburgh Medical Center (UPMC)-affiliated hospitals and its affiliated VA, VA

Box 2
Risk assessment index

1. Age, Sex, Cancer
   Sex Female = 0, Male = 5 _____
   Cancer (excluding nonmelanoma skin cancer) Score from Table below _____

| | Cancer | |
Age	No	Yes
<69	2	20
70–74	3	19
75–79	4	18
80–84	5	17
85–89	6	16
90–94	7	15
95–99	8	14
>100	9	13

2. Medical comorbidities "have you had:?" _____

Unintentional weight loss in 3 mo (>10 lbs)	5
Renal failure	6
Chronic/congestive heart failure	4
Poor appetite	4
Shortness of breath (at rest)	8

3. Activities of daily living and cognitive decline
   Mobility/eating/toileting/personal hygiene

For Each Category:

Independent	0
Supervised	1
Limited assistance	2
Extensive assistance	3
Total dependence	4

4. Add ADL scores and use table to find score

Without Cog Decline	With Cognitive Decline
1	−2
1,2	−1
3,4	0
5–7	+1
8,9	+2
10, 11	+3
12,13	+4
14–16 (max)	+5
Total Score	_____

Data from Hall DE, Arya S, Schmid KK, et al. Development and initial validation of the risk analysis index for measuring frailty in surgical populations. JAMA Surg 2017;152:175–82.

Pittsburgh. As of the authorship of this article, RAI scores on more than 100,000 patients have been accrued across the UPMC system. It is now a routine component of the preoperative evaluation of all surgical patients at UPMC (where it has been incorporated into the electronic medical record [EMR]) and at VA Pittsburgh. The clinical utility of this screening tool and how it drives additional evaluation and decision making are discussed in greater detail in the article on "Head and Neck Cancer in the Elderly" by Mady, and colleagues this issue. Outcome analysis of preoperative RAI scoring is currently driving modifications to the scoring schema with publication anticipated in the near future. Hopefully, implementation of the RAI will reduce the prevalence of low-value care in frail older adults.

The RAI-A was drawn from elements captured in 2 large surgical risk assessment databases, the VA Surgical Quality Improvement Project, and the ACS-NSQIP administered by the American College of Surgeons. The VA database was initially implemented more than 2 decades ago with the goal of comparing VA surgical care with civilian care. Although this goal was never achieved because of inadequate data from the non-VA sector, the project led to dramatic improvements in situational awareness for VA surgical leadership.[8] Risk-adjusted outcomes data were reported quarterly and have driven continuous and ongoing improvement in VA surgical care. Both risk assessment and outcomes data are generated through retrospective chart review by trained abstractors. Data on nearly 140 elements are collected. Audits have found high levels of reliability because of highly standardized data abstraction. Statistical calculations generate standardized risk assessment scores that are used to calculate expected 30-day mortality and morbidity rates. When compared with actual 30-day outcomes, data are reported as expected/outcomes ratio (OE ratio) for 30-day mortality or morbidity. OE ratios of less than 1 indicate better-than-expected outcomes, whereas ratios greater than 1 suggest poorer outcomes and the need for more careful examination. Although only specific surgical procedures are abstracted and uploaded to these databases, procedures conveying higher risk are selected and capped to achieve high levels of probabilistic accuracy. At the author's VA, approximately 30% of surgical cases are reviewed. This fact could potentially impact interpretation of NSQIP based retrospective studies.

AUTOMATED DATA EXTRACTION FROM ELECTRONIC MEDICAL RECORD

The data used in the RAI-A and the mFI are already present within the patient's EMR and theoretically could be extracted to construct a prospective risk assessment profile. A recent iteration of this strategy, the Rothman Index (RI)[9,10] is being used in several health care systems for inpatient risk assessment. The RI uses 26 data elements from 4 domains accessible within the EMR, including nursing observations, vital signs, cardiac rhythm, and laboratory tests. One can postulate that systems that have highly linked enterprisewide outpatient and inpatient EMR infrastructure may be able to implement new data mining paradigms, to include text-based phenotypic assessments, that may automate such prospective clinical decision support tools.

FRAILTY—SUMMARY

As of 2017 it appears we stand at the cusp of a widespread appreciation of the significance of frailty in diseases affecting older adults. The value of prospective measures of frailty that can assist in decision making will become even more apparent in coming years. It seems likely that geriatricians and others who specialize in the care of older adults will be called on to not only interpret numeric scores for specific patients, but also to contribute to the development and implementation of scoring measures. Geriatricians should take an active role in encouraging the health care systems in which they practice to select and standardize prospective assessment tools such as the RAI-C or similar easily administered measures. Further exploration of the utility of the RAI-C and similar risk assessment tools will undoubtedly add further support to the hypothesis that frailty is not only quantifiable, but that knowledge of its extent in specific patients can be used practically.

POLYPHARMACY

The impact of overmedication on the well-being of older adults is well recognized by geriatricians. As noted earlier, this level of understanding is not prevalent among nongeriatrician practitioners. This section of the article addresses recognized, and often unrecognized, manifestations of overmedication in older adults with otolaryngologic complaints.

Balance

Without question, the most common impact of overmedication in older adults is the impact on balance, predisposing affected patients to falls. This is discussed in some detail in the article on balance in this issue of *the Clinics*. The 2010 American Geriatric Society–British Geriatric Society Clinical Practice Guideline (AGS/BGS CPG) on Prevention of Falls is available at: http://www.geriatricscareonline.org/ProductAbstract/updated-american-geriatrics-societybritish-geriatrics-society-clinical-practice-guideline-for-prevention-of-falls-in-older-persons-and-recommendations/CL014 (Last accessed October 20, 2017). This document addresses the role of polypharmacy on fall risk, and places a high priority on reduction of medications, particularly psychoactive medications. A wide variety of medication classes can affect balance, including anticholinergics, antipsychotic medications, medications that induce orthostatic hypotension, and sleep aids. The reader is referred to the CPG document for more detailed information.[11]

Dysphagia

The effect of medications on swallowing function is often underappreciated. Otolaryngologists who evaluate patients with swallowing disorders often encounter patients with swallowing difficulties caused by diuretics, anticholinergics, or centrally acting sedatives. Because swallowing functional reserve decreases with increasing age (see the article on dysphagia in this issue of *the Clinics*) even minimal impairment of lubrication or motor coordination can tip relatively normal swallowing function into dysphagia. Xerostomia is a frequently encountered sequelae of taking medications with anticholinergic effects. A common offending medication in the elderly is oxybutynin-induced xerostomia, one of many commonly administered anticholinergics. The author advises his patients that "oxybutynin makes you dry below and also dry above," so the patient needs to decide whether staying dry below is important enough to warrant being dry above.

Reflux

Medications may affect gastroesophageal reflux (GER) and, in otolaryngology, extraesophageal reflux (often referred to as *laryngo-pharyngeal reflux*). Not only do some medications affect lower esophageal sphincter pressures, many common medications such as antihypertensive and cardiac medications also affect esophageal motility.[12] In addition to the effect on motility, anticholinergics and diuretics reduce salivary flow, so the normal rinsing and buffering effect of saliva on physiologic and pathologic GER is reduced. When combined with impairment of motility caused by aging, a common change accompanying aging, the effect of reflux is compounded.

Sinusitis and Postnasal Drip

There are no published studies correlating nasal and sinus complaints with medication usage, hence this paragraph should be interpreted as "expert opinion." All otolaryngologists encounter patients on a daily basis with complaints of sinus or postnasal drip, and these may be caused by medications. Anticholinergic and diuretic medications impair mucociliary function by reducing the sol layer of the mucus blanket. Reductions in this layer lead to ciliary dysfunction and mucus stasis. When this mucus reaches the posterior choana, it may adhere to the pharyngeal mucosa and be perceived as postnasal drip. A common observation by otolaryngologists is that patients who complain of postnasal drip typically have dry, adherent mucus rather than excessive amounts of mucus. Topical anticholinergic medications (ipratropium) are effective in reducing the copious amounts of clear nasal drainage in vasomotor rhinitis, often referred to as *senile drip*, but do not reduce symptoms for the patient with common sensation of postnasal drip. Moreover, treatment with antihistamines and nasal steroid sprays are often not beneficial and may even exacerbate symptoms and lead to bleeding because of the drying effect on nasal mucosa. It is worthwhile periodically stopping these medications as an empiric trial.

The turbinate nasal submucosa consists of a richly innervated vascular plexus. This plexus cycles through various stages of engorgement throughout the day. Medications that affect the autonomic nervous system, such as α-blockers, may impact the physiologic nasal cycle and lead to either increased obstruction or reduced turbinate volume precipitating excessive airflow and drying and crusting (and often bleeding).

There is general consensus by rhinologists, confirmed by the Cochrane Review,[13] that saline is an efficacious intervention for most symptomatic patients with dry nasal lining or thick mucus for whom medications cannot be eliminated. Environmental humidification is effective; however, saline instillation is the most effective way to moisturize the mucus blanket and assist in normalizing mucociliary function. Saline can be instilled by spray bottle or other device such as the "neti pot." The debate regarding isotonic, hypotonic, or hypertonic saline continues, but the optimal solution for most patients is to trial a few over-the-counter products, until they find the one that suits them best.

Summary of Polypharmacy in Otolaryngologic Diseases

Medications impact a wide range of medical disorders in the older adult, and many of these disorders fall within the category of otolaryngologic diseases. The effects of medications on balance are well known and outlined in detail in the 2010 AGS/BGS CPG on Falls. Less well known are the effects on xerostomia, with its attendant conditions such as burning mouth syndrome caused by loss of saliva and dysphagia. Inadequate salivary flow not only impairs oral function and swallowing but may also increase the symptomatic impact of gastroesophageal reflux. Finally, although no clinical trials exist to confirm the suspicion, many otolaryngologists suspect that medication-induced thickening and drying of nasal secretions may lead to the sensation of postnasal drip and an increased propensity for epistaxis.

The geriatric specialist is in a position to actively educate referring physicians as to the impact of polypharmacy. Alerting practitioners of other specialties to the challenge of polypharmacy and the existence of the Beer's criteria list may improve the quality of life for many older adults who are not under the care of a geriatrician. It is the opinion of this author that these educational efforts should also address the pharmacologic effects of medications with anticholinergic activity on the upper airway and swallowing passages.

REFERENCES

1. Makary MA, Segev DL, Pronovost PJ, et al. Frailty as a predictor of surgical outcomes in older patients. J Am Coll Surg 2010;210:901–8.
2. Adams P, Ghanem T, Stachler R, et al. Frailty as a predictor of morbidity and mortality in inpatient head and neck surgery. JAMA Otolaryngol Head Neck Surg 2013;138:783–9.
3. Revenig LM, Canter DJ, Taylor MD, et al. Too frail for surgery? Initial results of a large multidisciplinary prospective study examining preoperative variables predictive of poor surgical outcomes. J Am Coll Surg 2013;217:665–70.
4. Selb CD, Rochefort H, Chromsky-Higgins K, et al. Association of patient frailty with increased morbidity after common ambulatory general surgery operations. JAMA Surg 2017. Available at: https://jamanetwork.com/journals/jamasurgery/article-abstract/2656841?redirect=true. Accessed October 20, 2017.
5. Dent E, Kowal P, Hoogendijk EO. Frailty measurement in research and clinical practice: a review. Eur J Intern Med 2016;31:3–10.
6. Frailty assessment tool. Available at: http://geriatricscareonline.org/SearchResult/index/index/category_name/Frailty. Accessed October 20, 2017.
7. Hall DE, Arya S, Schmid KK, et al. Development and initial validation of the risk analysis index for measuring frailty in surgical populations. JAMA Surg 2017; 152:175–82.
8. Khuri SF, Jennifer Daley J, Henderson W, et al. The Department of Veterans Affairs' NSQIP: the first national, validated, outcome-based, risk-adjusted, and peer-controlled program for the measurement and enhancement of the quality of surgical care. Ann Surg 1998;228:491–507.
9. Rothman MJ, Rothman SI, Beals J 4th. Development and validation of a continuous measure of patient condition using the electronic medical record. J Biomed Inform 2013;48:837–48.
10. Tepas JJ, Rimar JM, Hsiao AL, et al. Automated analysis of electronic medical record data reflects the pathophysiology of operative complications. Surgery 2013; 154:918–26.
11. American Geriatrics Society (AGS) and British Geriatrics Society (BGS) panel on the clinical practice guideline for the prevention of falls in older persons. AGS/BGS clinical practice guideline: prevention of falls in older persons. 2010. Available at: http://www.geriatricscareonline.org/ProductAbstract/updated-american-geriatrics-societybritish-geriatrics-society-clinical-practice-guideline-for-prevention-of-falls-in-older-persons-and-recommendations/CL014. Accessed October 20, 2017.
12. Tutuian R. Adverse effects of drugs on the esophagus. Best Pract Res Clin Gastroenterol 2010;24:91–7.
13. Chong LY, Head K, Hopkins C, et al. Saline irrigation for chronic rhinosinusitis. Cochrane Database Syst Rev 2016;26:4.

Moving?

Make sure your subscription moves with you!

To notify us of your new address, find your **Clinics Account Number** (located on your mailing label above your name), and contact customer service at:

Email: journalscustomerservice-usa@elsevier.com

800-654-2452 (subscribers in the U.S. & Canada)
314-447-8871 (subscribers outside of the U.S. & Canada)

Fax number: 314-447-8029

Elsevier Health Sciences Division
Subscription Customer Service
3251 Riverport Lane
Maryland Heights, MO 63043

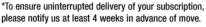

Moving?

Make sure your subscription moves with you!

To notify us of your new address, find your Clinics Account Number (located on your mailing label above your name), and contact customer service at:

Email: JournalsCustomerService-usa@elsevier.com

800-654-2452 (subscribers in the U.S. & Canada)
314-447-8871 (subscribers outside of the U.S. & Canada)

Fax number: 314-447-8029

Elsevier Health Sciences Division
Subscription Customer Service
3251 Riverport Lane
Maryland Heights, MO 63043

To ensure uninterrupted delivery of your subscription, please notify us at least 4 weeks in advance of move.

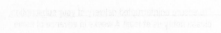

Printed and bound by CPI Group (UK) Ltd, Croydon, CR0 4YY

03/10/2024

01040395-0015